Mindfulness For Insomnia

A Four-Week Guided Program To Relax Your Body, Calm Your Mind, And Get The Sleep You Need
Catherine Polan Orzech, MA, LMFT
William H. Moorcroft, PhD

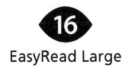

EasyRead Large

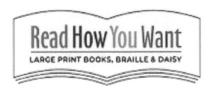

Read How You Want
LARGE PRINT BOOKS, BRAILLE & DAISY

Copyright Page from the Original Book

Publisher's Note

Distributed in Canada by Raincoast Books

Copyright © 2019 by William M. Moorcroft and Catherine Polan Orzech
New Harbinger Publications, Inc.
5674 Shattuck Avenue
Oakland, CA 94609
www.newharbinger.com

The exercise "Three-Minute Breathing Space" is adapted from *Mindfulness-Based Cognitive Therapy for Depression* by Zindel V. Segal, J. Mark G. Williams, and John D. Teasdale. © 2002 Guilford Press. Used by permission.

The exercises "Affectionate Breathing," "How Do You Treat a Friend," and "Self-Compassion Break" are adapted from the *Mindful Self-Compassion Workbook* by Kristin Neff and Christopher Germer. © 2018 Guilford Press. Used by permission.

Rumi, excerpt from "The Guesthouse," translated by Coleman Barks. Copyright © 1997 by Coleman Barks. Used by permission.

Cover design by Amy Daniel; Text design by Michele Waters and Tracy Carlson; Acquired by Wendy Millstine;Edited by Ken Knabb;

Library of Congress Cataloging-in-Publication Data on file

21   20   19

10   9   8   7   6   5   4   3   2   1   First Printing

TABLE OF CONTENTS

"*Mindfulness for Insomnia* is an in-depth guide to mindfulness and compassion training, as well as to the science of sleep. The book offers a dynamic combination of invaluable information and practical skills to support mind and body wellness. I highly recommend the four-week GMATI program skillfully detailed in this book for anyone who wants to reduce stress and improve sleep."

—**Diane Reibel, PhD,** director of the Myrna Brind Center for Mindfulness at Thomas Jefferson University Hospitals, coauthor of *Teaching Mindfulness,* and coeditor of *Resources for Teaching Mindfulness*

"As a busy person who struggles with insomnia, I found *Mindfulness for Insomnia* to be a practical and accessible guide toward better sleep. As a mindfulness practitioner for over fifteen years and a member of Thich Nhat Hanh's Plumb Village for a year, I consider its approach to mindfulness practice to be spot-on. And as a human in our complex and often chaotic world, this book helped me manage stress, find greater acceptance, and manage daily suffering from chronic illness with greater ease, and even joy. *Mindfulness for Insomnia* is packed with excellent meditation techniques. It is a practical and thorough guide, not only to sleeping better but also to living a healthier life. I highly recommend it."

—**Courtney Zenner Campbell,** studied Buddhist philosophy intensively in college (in addition to practicing Buddhism since 2004), has taken a mindfulness-based stress reduction (MBSR) course, and was a resident at Thich Nhat Hanh's Plumb Village for a year

"This book is a comprehensive guidebook and resource to get back to regular and restful sleep. Catherine Polan Orzech and Bill Moorcroft have pulled from a wide range of practices, disciplines, and subject matter, as well as a wealth of professional experience between them, to inform and teach useful life and sleep practices. The progression of guided exercises is straightforward and supported as if you are being personally coached along the way. Enjoy the richness of learning provided in this book and be well!"

—Deanna O'Connell, is a mindfulness practitioner in Fort Collins, CO

"Catherine Polan Orzech and William Moorcroft do an excellent job bringing what can be a complicated but extremely effective treatment for insomnia into an easy-to-read format. It is fortunate that now many people suffering from insomnia, who may not be able to access therapists trained in this technique, can now follow step-by-step instructions through this book. This guide consists of well-formulated, day-to-day instructions paired with online meditation recordings to provide a road map for those struggling with insomnia and desiring a behavioral approach that lasts long term."

—**Nicole Cirino, MD,** reproductive psychiatrist, and associate professor and director of the Women's Mental Health and Wellness Program at the Center for Women's Health at Oregon Health & Science University

"*Mindfulness for Insomnia* outlines a four-week program that provides people suffering from insomnia with a gentle method to work with their sleep-disrupting thoughts. Using a series of mindfulness practices and important information about how our minds can impact our sleep, the reader learns and uses daily mindfulness practice to move away from the insomnia struggle and in the direction of calm, restful sleep."

—**Jennifer L. Martin, PhD,** is a clinical psychologist and academic researcher in Los Angeles, CA. She is associate professor of medicine at the University of California, Los Angeles

"Thanks for an incredible treatment option for those suffering from insomnia! Although cognitive behavioral therapy for insomnia (CBT-I) is very effective, it does not work for everybody. *Mindfulness for Insomnia* offers an alternate approach to treatment which helps disarm the fears and anxiety so many with insomnia experience. I am grateful to have this book as a resource for my patients!"

—**Ryan Wetzler, PsyD, DBSM, ABPP,** founder of Sleep Health Center in Louisville, KY; and codeveloper of Night Owl-Sleep Coach, a CBT-I-based insomnia treatment app

"If you find yourself trying harder and harder to overcome your insomnia, you may be discovering that it becomes more and more difficult to sleep. The dilemma of insomnia is beautifully articulated (and solved) in this informative, practical, and clear guide to bringing mindfulness to our challenges with sleep. Written in a light and inspiring style, this excellent book draws on the deep wisdom of mindfulness and compassion to support you in moving beyond insomnia. Let psychologists and mindfulness teachers, Catherine Polan Orzech and Bill Moorcroft, gently guide you to finding ease and sleep through the meditative practices of mindfulness and compassion, and maybe find some new ways to contend with stress of all sorts in your life."

—**Steven D. Hickman, PsyD,** clinical psychologist and executive director at the Center for Mindful Self-Compassion, founding director of the UC San Diego Center for Mindfulness, and associate clinical professor at the UC San Diego School of Medicine

Acknowledgments

CATHERINE POLAN ORZECH:

To Wendy Millstine of New Harbinger, who eight years ago reached out to me and asked if I'd write a book about mindfulness. I am grateful that she persisted. To Ryan Buresh and Caleb Beckwith, thank you for being patient and creative editors who helped shape how these teachings could best reach readers.

Without the hundreds of people who have attended the MBSR and MSC and other mindfulness classes I've taught over the last twenty years, and the many clients who have come through my practice seeking a deeper healing connection to themselves, this book would not have been possible. What I have learned through sitting with all these people humbles me and inspires my belief in the healing power of a mind infused with mindful awareness and loving-kindness.

With the most humble and profound gratitude, I want to thank my teachers who have shared the wisdom of the dharma with me and embodied compassionate mindful awareness. To the many vipassana meditation teachers who have led retreats I have attended, to Jon Kabat-Zinn, who has tirelessly pioneered the dissemination of mindfulness, to Kristin Neff and Chris Germer, who developed the mindful self-compassion program and who persist in exploring and teaching compassion, I offer my endless gratitude. To Steve Hickman, the traveling bodhisattva: You inspire me by your endless ability to teach and share with more loving connected presence than seems humanly possible. And to Diane Reibel, my mentor and my friend: Without you and your guidance in meditation and in teaching, I would not be where I am today. I owe you more than I can possibly say. Thank you!

To my dear, dear friends Ilyana Karthas and Doris Ferleger: You have been constant inspirations. To Jessica Landry, who believed in my ability to write long before I ever thought it was possible. And to Michelle Kalman: The myriad hours you spent patiently listening and reflecting are invaluable. To all of you, I offer my thanks.

To Bill Moorcroft, who courageously went on this journey with me. Thank you for being my accomplice!

To my parents, my endless supporters, with loving thanks!

To Rafael Orzech, who is my biggest fan, and to Dan Orzech, thank you for sharing me with this long process and for always holding things together. I love you both!

WILLIAM H. MOORCROFT:

First and foremost, I want to acknowledge how grateful I am to my life-mate, Laurie Dunn. It is amazing that this late in our lives we found each other and enjoy each other so much. Laurie was enormously patient and understanding every time I returned to the computer to "work on the book." And she was always willing to listen to me talk about "how the book is going," and to pitch in to do the things around the house that "I did not have time to do." Life with her is a wonderful thing.

I would also like to express my gratitude to Jason Ong for encouraging me to proceed with writing this book and for helping guide me to its publisher, New Harbinger.

This book would not have come to fruition without the cooperation of numerous clients over several years, who helped me hone GMATI as I used a progression of versions on them. Thanks to you all.

Like Catherine, I also give a shout-out to the folks at New Harbinger who helped get Catherine and me together to write this book, and for their continued help and guidance along the way as the project proceeded.

Foreword

Sleep is easy. You get into bed, turn off the lights, close your eyes, and blissfully drift off to sleep. About seven to eight hours later, you wake up feeling refreshed and ready to take on the world. This is how sleep is *supposed* to happen, right?

Unfortunately, many people find that sleep does not happen this way on most nights. About one-third of adults experience some difficulty falling or staying asleep, and about ten to fifteen percent of adults suffer from chronic insomnia. If you are one of the millions who suffer from insomnia, you have probably found sleep to be effortful and unpredictable, and you might have lost confidence in your ability to sleep. You have probably heard of sleep hygiene and have tried following all of the rules to a tee, but this hasn't solved your sleep problem. Desperate for some relief, you might have turned to sleep medications to help knock you out, only to find that you now worry about dependence and long-term use. Sound familiar?

Fortunately, there is an approach that can improve the quality of your sleep *and* the quality of your wakefulness, without drugs or a list of sleep hygiene rules. It is called mindfulness meditation. Although mindfulness meditation is relatively new to Western society, it is actually not a new approach but one that is rooted in the philosophy and practice of Buddhism. Programs teaching the principles and practices of mindfulness meditation have been developed to help people who are suffering from chronic health conditions such as insomnia. There is now a substantial body of research evidence demonstrating the health benefits of mindfulness meditation across a number of different chronic conditions including coping with symptoms of cancer, preventing the relapse of depression, and reducing symptoms of anxiety. Several randomized controlled trials have been conducted on people with sleep disturbances, showing that mindfulness programs have a significant impact on reducing insomnia symptoms and improving sleep quality.

So why isn't everybody with insomnia practicing mindfulness meditation? First of all, access to a mindfulness program can be difficult. Although the number is growing, there is still a limited number of places that offer mindfulness programs. Second, mindfulness is not as easy as taking medications, and primary care physicians are generally not used to recommending meditation programs as a way to help their patients. Finally, some people have the perception that meditation is only for religious purposes—not something that can improve their health.

That's where this book comes in. This book is not for monks nor people with special training in meditation or religion. There are no tricks or gimmicks for falling asleep faster, and no short-cuts for solving your sleep problems. What this book has to offer are techniques grounded in mindfulness meditation that can help connect your mind, body, and spirit to this moment so that sleep will come back and find you. Catherine Orzech and Bill Moorcroft have put together a four-week program called GMATI, which uses mindfulness practices, self-compassion training, and acceptance techniques to help reduce the effort and anxiety about trying to make sleep happen. They will teach you how to bring mindfulness practices into your everyday life, providing instructions to lead you every step of the way. It is packed with information on the biology of sleep, the principles of mindfulness meditation, and guided meditations to help establish your meditation practice. From basic tips to common struggles, their pointers will help the novice meditator feel comfortable with starting a mindfulness meditation practice. By bringing in self-compassion, they also teach you how to be kind and loving towards yourself—something that is very easy to forget when we are tired and just want some rest. What is particularly creative and interesting about this program is that they barely mention any instructions or rules for what to do at night! Instead, they teach you how to focus on improving the quality of your wakefulness so that you can sleep better at night. This makes sense because insomnia is a problem where the harder you try to fix it, the more you become stuck in a vicious cycle.

This book is for anyone who is interested in learning about mindfulness and who is willing to put in the work to practice mindfulness meditation. Whether you are just starting your journey into mindfulness or you are looking for a way to reinforce your meditation practice, this book will be a valuable companion. For the clinician who works with insomnia patients, there are resources to provide guidance for using these techniques to enhance your clinical practice.

Practicing mindfulness meditation takes time and patience. It's not easy. But you might discover that letting go of how sleep is *supposed* to be is the first step toward improving your sleep health.

—Jason C. Ong, PhD,

Author of *Mindfulness-Based Therapy for Insomnia*

Introduction

Welcome to *Mindfulness for Insomnia!* If you have purchased or picked up this book, it is likely because you have been suffering—suffering from the grief, stress, frustration, exhaustion, mental fogginess, and perhaps even despair that come from insomnia. We want you to know right from the start that we honor and recognize the courage it takes to pick up yet another book and try again. By reading this book and engaging in the practices that we will be teaching you, you are beginning a journey. And as the pithy saying goes, each journey begins with just one step.

You've made that step and we will be with you every subsequent step on the way. We've designed this book to walk with you daily for four weeks. But before we get into how this book is structured, we want to introduce ourselves so you know who you have with you.

For years, both of us have been treating people just like you who suffer from insomnia, each in our own way. Dr. Bill Moorcroft comes from a background in researching, writing, and teaching about sleep. Catherine Polan Orzech is a therapist experienced in teaching, researching, and doing presentations about mindfulness—particularly mindfulness-based stress reduction (MBSR) and mindful self-compassion (MSC). From these different backgrounds, both of us have come to understand the incredible value mindfulness meditation has to offer people struggling with insomnia.

Meet Bill:

Bill's background is a more traditional route to working with insomnia. Since retiring from his position teaching and researching sleep at Luther College (Decorah, Iowa) in 2002, he's been using the standard cognitive behavioral therapy for insomnia (CBTI) and has treated over 400 patients with this method. But that approach changed the day a married couple, Joe and Susan, came in for treatment. (All the names of patients mentioned in this book have been changed to protect their privacy.) As was his customary approach, he began the treatment using CBTI to help them directly make changes to improve their sleep. Both Joe and Susan were in the room at the same time, and received exactly the same information and instructions. However, after a couple of sessions it was obvious that while Joe's sleep had begun to improve, Susan's sleep was getting worse. When Dr. Moorcroft asked her about this, she said that because of directly focusing on her sleep and trying to do things to improve it (as prescribed by CBTI) she had actually become more anxious about sleep, which made her sleep worse. This in turn made her even more anxious, which was ruining her sleep even further. She was in a downward spiral.

Around this same time, Bill had been reading published reports by Dr. Jason Ong and other sleep experts (Ong and Sholtes, 2010) about how they were beginning to use mindfulness meditation to treat groups of people who complained of insomnia. He immediately switched Susan's treatment to guided mindfulness meditation. She grabbed hold of it and, lo and behold, it worked: she reported that her sleep quickly got better.

Following this success, Dr. Moorcroft worked at developing a systematic sequence of mindfulness practices to help people suffering from insomnia on an individual basis. The result is a new four-session protocol for individuals called Guided Mindfulness with Acceptance Treatment for Insomnia (GMATI), which he has since been using to successfully treat the many people seeking relief from the suffering of insomnia.

Now meet Catherine:

Catherine Polan Orzech's story is quite different. In 1997, Catherine was introduced to the mindfulness-based stress reduction (MBSR) program. This program had been developed by Jon Kabat-Zinn in 1979 at the University of Massachusetts Medical Center as a treatment for patients with severe chronic pain. Because of its success, the type of patients who were referred to the program expanded beyond those experiencing chronic pain to all different types of maladies. The program wasn't there to treat the diseases themselves, but to help people change their relationship to the suffering they were experiencing—which often helped with whatever the underlying illness was. Catherine initially went to this program not as a clinician, but as a patient. After a brief career as a professional ballet dancer (and then a switch to social work and marriage and family therapy), Catherine was suffering from some significant health crises of her own, and the program was recommended to her to help her cope. Learning mindfulness meditation not only helped her cope, it significantly reduced the symptoms she was experiencing. It then became her life's work.

Catherine devoted herself to a daily meditation practice and also attended meditation retreats to deepen that practice. She began sharing what she was learning with her own clients, and then in 2004, was trained and later certified to teach mindfulness-based stress reduction. Catherine has taught in some of the country's leading health institutions. Just as with the University of Massachusetts Medical Center program, the participants in the MBSR groups she taught were experiencing major medical crises—cancer, heart disease, orthopedic traumas, diabetes, chronic pain, and so forth, as well as emotional sufferings such as depression, anxiety, and grief. Even though insomnia was not what they listed as their primary concern, it was frequently a co-occurring problem. This was also true with the clients she was working with individually in therapy. Catherine rarely directly approached the sleep issues, or the cancers or heart disease or other health problems, as the focus of the class or individual treatment. She was there to share with them the practice of mindfulness, and to help people reconnect with their wholeness beyond whatever illnesses or difficulties were plaguing their bodies and emotions. But even though insomnia wasn't directly addressed, it almost always improved. And for those whose sleep didn't actually change, they suffered less because they weren't struggling with it anymore. This freed them up to seek other resources, as well as to embrace the life they did have. And that made people a lot happier.

Later, in 2014, Catherine was introduced to the work of Kristin Neff and her research on mindful self-compassion, and this became another pivotal experience that she could offer to the people in her classes and clinic. Compassion had always been a part of her teaching in mindfulness, but with a deeper understanding of how to skillfully apply it to oneself—which is what the mindful self-compassion program is all about—she saw even greater benefits in how suffering could be alleviated in the people she was working with. Catherine was thus also trained and then later certified to teach the mindful self-compassion program. She has seen tremendous benefit in helping people develop a kinder relationship to themselves.

Both of us are thrilled to share how to use guided mindfulness to improve your sleep. That's why we teamed up to write this book for you and others suffering with insomnia. Coming from our different backgrounds, each of us brings knowledge and skills that complement one another. The result is optimal GMATI effectiveness. We now want to share this approach for treating people on an individual basis who suffer from insomnia because of anxiety or for whom the traditional CBTI does not seem appropriate or has been unsuccessful.

Now about you:

You may be like most people who suffer from chronic insomnia, who describe their condition as being caught in a "vicious cycle" of poor sleep, which triggers concern, which in turn causes more poor sleep, which results in even more concern, and so on. Many of them also find that the increasing effort and desire they put into trying to improve their sleep only seems to make it worse, not better. Their struggles with unwanted thoughts, emotions, and physical sensations associated with insomnia increase physiological arousal levels, which perpetuate their sleeplessness. The result is frustration, stress, and especially anxiety, which interferes with their sleep even more. Directly trying to change their sleep, such as by using CBTI, may be unsuccessful for such people. Instead, they need to let go of directly trying to "fix" their sleep. Does this sound like you?

If it does, this book may be just what you need.

Here's how you can get the most out of this book. Part 1 ("Understanding the Fundamentals") will introduce you to what we think the problem really is. You'll find out about mindfulness and then learn some things about sleep itself that can beneficially correct several common misconceptions.

In part 2 ("The Practicals of Practice"), you will learn about the GMATI approach. We will guide you day by day in how to practice mindfulness. Each of the four weeks will have a new guided meditation recording, which you can access and download from the New Harbinger website—http://www.newharbinger.com/425 87. (See the very back of this book for more details on accessing these recordings and other materials that you can use for your practice.) The GMATI meditation practices have been specifically designed for people struggling with insomnia. In each weekly chapter, the theme for the week will be introduced, and then you will have a short reading for each day and suggestions for how you can deepen your practice and get the most out of it. You will also be introduced to additional guided meditations that come from Catherine's long experience of teaching programs like MBSR and mindful self-compassion, as well as wisdom gleaned from the great lineage of Western meditation masters. And so, you, too, will get to experience some of the elements of those programs that will support and supplement the GMATI meditations. We hope that you will feel like you are being personally coached through these practices as we "sit" with you every day.

It can be tempting to rush on ahead and maybe even double up days. But it is really better to just read each day's entry one day at a time and then practice each and every day. You will get much more out of doing it daily then saving it all up for one day.

We look forward to being with you through this process. Let's begin!

The information and resources in this book are sufficient for you to use the GMATI approach to improve your sleep. They can also be used by clinicians for adoption of GMATI as a part of their practice for treating individuals with insomnia (see supplement for clinicians on the New Harbinger website: http://www.newharbinger.com/42587).

PART 1

Understanding the Fundamentals

CHAPTER 1

Why We Have Trouble Sleeping

You're not sleeping and you feel miserable all day because of it. Your brain is foggy and you can't concentrate. Your work and relationships are suffering. You feel helpless and hopeless and worry that you may never sleep again. Wanting to feel rested and being unable to have taken over every aspect of your life. But you haven't been able to change this. Sleeping pills are not working or maybe you just do not want to have to keep taking them anymore. (Note: If wanting or needing to get off sleeping pills is your problem, we ask you to be patient. You will need to acquire things that will replace what the sleeping pills are doing for you before you give them up. GMATI can do that, but first you have to do the whole GMATI program. In the last chapter of this book, we will show you how you can taper off of sleeping pills with the support of GMATI.)

In this chapter, we'll introduce you to a refreshingly new, encouraging, and empowering understanding of how your perception of and your reactions to your insomnia—usually in the form of resistance—lock you into a negative cycle, the continuation of your insomnia, and add to your suffering.

First, let's look at some people who, just like you, struggled with insomnia and sought help through mindfulness.

Cynthia sat in the first session of the mindfulness-based stress reduction (MBSR) class she had registered for and laughed nervously as she introduced herself. "I'm having one of those 'power surges' right now," she said as she wiped the hot flash-induced sweat from her brow and tried to fan herself with the binder she had received for the class. "I'm here because I feel angry all the time that these hormonal changes are happening and I can't enjoy my life. I'm exhausted and that makes me snap at my husband and kids, and then I feel really bad about myself." Her intake paperwork revealed that she was waking up in the middle of the night and that she would toss and turn for a while and then just get up because she was so frustrated. Sometimes she would wander into the kitchen and eat because she didn't know what else to do. Her mind would race and her body felt agitated and restless. "I'm really ashamed that I don't have more self-control. But I just can't shut my mind off. My body will feel all flooded with heat and then my legs feel restless. I just have to get up. But then I think about how I'm going to get through the next day and I just can't bear lying there anymore. Eating gives me something to do, but then I just feel bad. When I try to lay back down and go to sleep, all I can think about is how stupid I am for all that I ate, and how my life is unraveling."

Sam registered for an MBSR class because his oncologist had heard that mindfulness could be helpful in working with his pain. He was skeptical that meditating could really help him, but since he'd tried everything else, he figured he had nothing to lose. The chronic nerve pain had started after his radiation therapy for prostate cancer three years ago. "Without heavy-duty pain meds, I haven't been able to sit comfortably, never mind sleep, in all that time," he reported. He became teary as he talked about how he felt like he was losing his life to pain and to feeling mentally and physically exhausted all the time because he couldn't sleep. "I just have no hope that I'll ever enjoy my life again. I really believe I'll never be able to sleep or be comfortable in my body again."

Alex worked as an accountant. He had always been healthy and able to push himself to his limits physically and mentally. He prided himself on needing only a few hours of sleep at night, so he could work late into the night and then wake up early to work out. "But recently," he says, "When I want to sleep, I can't. It's like I can't shut off. I used to be able to control it, but not anymore. I'm getting more and more irritable and I hate myself for it. My wife has asked me to sleep in another room because I'm waking her up with all my agitation. I'm afraid if I don't get a handle on myself it's going to have a bad impact on my marriage."

You, dear reader, like the people in the examples above, are not alone. Nearly a quarter of the population says they struggle with sleep. This increases to about one-third in the elderly. And more than one out of ten people of any age have chronic insomnia: they have trouble sleeping at least three nights a week, for periods of three months or longer. Some of them have trouble falling asleep (called sleep-onset insomnia). Others sleep soundly for a few hours but then wake up and then have difficulty sustaining sleep (called sleep-maintenance insomnia). Still others may awaken too early in the morning and are unable to return to sleep (called early arousal insomnia). Many people suffer from one or a combination of these types of insomnia or shift from one type to another over time. Can you relate your sleep problem to these types?

Actually, there are numerous reasons why you may have some type of insomnia. They can range from hormonal and biological fluctuations, to chronic pain, to stress in your waking life, to anxiety, to simple habits that are interfering with the basic sleep mechanisms, among others. Each of these situations is a challenge in and of itself. Add in the resulting insomnia and you have a lot of suffering!

This book addresses what most other books on insomnia do not: the "mental threats" that both feed and keep you stuck in patterns of insomnia (which add even more suffering). That's what mindfulness and self-compassion can help with, and that is what this book is about.

There is nothing you can do to "make" yourself sleep. If you've ever lain awake telling yourself, *Go to sleep, go to sleep,* or even conjured up images of nineteenth-century hypnotists waving golden pocket watches in front of your eyes intoning those same words, all to no avail, you know that to be true. In many ways, this is why this condition can be so maddening. In fact, the more you try to bully yourself into going to sleep and tell yourself to do it, the more your mind and your body seem to rebel. If you've ever lain down with a toddler trying to wait them out at a scheduled naptime, you know. No amount of wishing, commanding, or pleading can "make" the child fall asleep. What you can do, however, is to create the conditions, internally and externally, to tip the scales and make sleep more likely to happen when you do lie down. You can *allow* sleep to come by working with your mind and your body.

Resistance: The Second Arrow

Here's a formula for suffering: Suffering = Pain x Resistance. "Pain" in this formula equals difficulty—like the difficulty of sleeplessness. You can think of "resistance" as the thoughts and feelings you have when you can't sleep (or when you experience anything that you don't want to be happening). It's the *reactivity* to something unwanted. Experiencing "resistance" can include a racing mind, anxiety, grief, hopelessness, helplessness, or perhaps idealistic expectations of sleep.

Working with the mind often means working with resistance. All of us naturally put up resistance to whatever we perceive as causing us to suffer. To be very clear, understanding how you might be resisting should *not* be just another way to blame yourself for the situation you're in. All of us are fundamentally programmed to want things to be different from how they are when we are feeling pain or discomfort. So of course we are resistant to feeling exhausted!

It's extremely uncomfortable to be exhausted and feel like your brain and body can't function. Not sleeping sucks. But here's the surprising part: whenever we are continually grasping after a reality that is different from the one we are actually in, or actively resisting our current experience, we inadvertently create an increase in anxiety, an increase in stress, an increase in grief, an increase in fear, an increase in helplessness, and an increase in hopelessness. All these agitated states tell the body that there is some kind of crisis, and then, as a way of trying to reregulate and protect itself, our bodies go into fight/flight mode, which makes sleep even more elusive. We get ourselves into a loop of suffering that just compounds upon itself. It's a vicious cycle.

Take, for example, when your mind is overactive. This can bring an agitated energy to your body, which you experience as restlessness. The restlessness then makes your mind start spinning more about how uncomfortable things are, triggering desperation to try to fix the problem—which in turn creates more tension in your body. Round and round it goes! This is the epitome of a vicious cycle. There is very little chance here for you to be able to enter into a state of relaxation where sleep can take hold.

There's a story that comes out of Buddhist teachings that describes how easily we can inadvertently cause a lot of our own suffering and find ourselves in this vicious cycle. The metaphor in the story is called "the second arrow." In this particular teaching, the Buddha asks: "If you get struck by an arrow, do you then shoot another arrow into yourself?"

We can consider the factors of biology, stress, and the like as the first arrow. Things happen and our bodies react. This happens in a moment and creates a certain result. What you do from there, the reactivity you go into—ruminating on the situation, making lists of strategies to fix things, blaming yourself, others, and everything wrong in your life—that's the second arrow. That's the part you add. That's the proliferation of thoughts and subsequent emotions that only turn up the dial on your experience of suffering and sleeplessness. These thoughts and emotions consume a lot of energy and exacerbate the next day's negative consequences of poor sleep.

Understanding Stress

When we're talking about "suffering," we are also talking about *stress.* Your internally programmed stress-response system gets turned on whenever your mind is saying, "There's something wrong here!" To understand a little bit more of how that works, let's first look at a definition of stress paraphrased from Stanford neuroendocrinologist Robert Sapolsky in his groundbreaking book *Why Zebras Don't Get Ulcers* (1998). Simply put, *stress is the perception of a threat to one's physical or psychological well-being, coupled with the belief that you can't handle the situation.*

What's important to look at first is that it starts with *perception.* This is really important, because once you are mindfully aware of your perceptions, you can change your relationship to them. How you see or perceive things determines the thoughts, emotions, body sensations, and even behaviors that follow. In order to understand that more directly, try this experiment:

Imagine you are walking down a busy street. There are people all around you, and on the opposite side of the street, you see someone you know. In your exuberance to connect, you throw up your hand and start waving madly and calling out that person's name. But that person keeps walking and doesn't acknowledge you at all.

Now, pause. Notice what thoughts or reactions may be running through your mind. Notice what emotions you may be experiencing. And notice how your body feels.

Depending on your *perception* of what's happening, you could have a variety of reactions. Some common responses are feelings of embarrassment, anger, and insecurity. But some people may feel that "everything is fine." The people who report experiencing embarrassment say that they are aware of having thoughts like, *I must look so stupid! What was I thinking to make such a scene?* They even say that just imagining this scenario causes their bodies to feel hot and flushed, with a creeping of adrenaline up their chest and neck.

Those who say they feel insecure report that they have thoughts like, *Is he mad at me? Did I do something wrong for him to ignore me?* They may also say they feel tension in their chest and their hearts are beating a little faster. The folks who say they feel angry say they have blaming thoughts like, *What's wrong with her?!* Increased body tension goes along with that one, too. The people who report feeling fine state that the thoughts they had were, *Maybe she didn't see me.* Or, *It must have been someone else.* They don't report experiencing any increase in tension. So you can see that different perceptions of the situation determined how different people experienced it, psychologically and physiologically.

Sometimes, even not getting sleep can be perceived as "not a problem." Imagine that you are heading out for a weeklong beach vacation. You have been looking forward to this trip for a long time. The flight to get you there leaves at 6:30a.m., which means you need to be at the airport at 5:00. You set your alarm for 4:00 so that you will have time to get dressed, get to the airport, park the car, and make it through the security lines. You may feel tired; you may even feel foggy-headed and slow. But usually the enthusiasm and excitement (which in part caused you to get less sleep) carry you through. In other words, you have framed getting less sleep as "not a problem" in this situation.

In most situations, however, we experience not sleeping as a major problem. And along with the experience or perception of "problem" come difficult sensations in the body and mind. One really amazing thing is that these feelings and body sensations can arise when all we are doing is sitting in a room and just imagining this scenario! Our minds are incredibly powerful, and the type of thinking we are experiencing, based on our initial perceptions, can determine what we feel and how our bodies react. We can turn on our own stress response simply by thinking about something distressing.

The other thing about Sapolsky's work on stress that is really interesting is that he indicates that it's a perception of a *threat* to our physical or psychological well-being. Our threat-detection system is well developed, but it's not very sophisticated. The part of the reptilian brain, called the amygdala, that does this job can't tell the difference between a physical threat, like a fierce predator, or a psychological threat, such as a threat to our sense of self. These psychological threats can be things like running late, forgetting to send an email, or believing you may fail at your job because you are tired and foggy-headed again. It's like having a dinosaur in charge of how you see the world. The dinosaur can't distinguish between a saber-toothed tiger threat and a simply-being-worried threat. It initiates a chain of physiological reactions that are aimed at survival. These physiological reactions are an outpouring of adrenaline and cortisol, tightening of the muscles, increase of heart rate and respirations, blood flow being diverted to the large muscles, and less access to your prefrontal cortex to do rational thinking. These reactions are all completely necessary if you need to fight for your life, run away from an oncoming bus, or freeze and play dead so the large predator won't eat you. It's great that we have a system that is such an internal bodyguard, but it can be a little hyperreactive. Imagine having a bodyguard detail that pulled out its guns every time you got a text message that made you think someone was mad at you, or even every time you were mad at yourself and saying nasty things to yourself in your own mind. We'd say, *Dude! Chill out. Learn some discernment!*

In our modern life, the stress response gets a real workout because of chronic activation. The days can feel like they tumble from one threat to the next and the system never gets a break. And remember, we can turn on our own stress response simply by telling ourselves, *I can't do this! I'm going to die because I'm so tired!*

That initial appraisal of "problem," regardless of what the problem is, whom it is aimed at, and where it comes from, ignites this well-designed survival mechanism. Learning how to slow down and be aware of the thoughts that go into that initial appraisal is essential to dialing down the stress response system and therefore the suffering that can come from it.

Now, this system is hard-wired and we need it. It is there for our survival and is one of the branches of our autonomic nervous system (ANS), which is responsible for biological functions. This branch is called the SNS or sympathetic nervous system. The other branch of the ANS is the para-sympathetic nervous system (PNS), also called the calm and connection response or the relaxation response. We are designed to have the PNS turned on most of the time, while the purpose of the SNS is to respond to emergencies and help us survive.

Styles of Thinking

We just saw how what we are perceiving and therefore thinking can have powerful effects on our stress responses. We also saw that not everybody thinks and reacts the same. A major reason for this is differences in our styles of thinking. Our ways of thinking are conditionally developed—genetics, experiences, and beliefs all play a role in our styles of thinking.

Our thoughts show up in the form of images as well as narratives. Like clouds, they can have all sorts of intensities and configurations. Some are light and wispy and barely noticeable. Others are compelling, commanding our attention and refusing to let us go. Some thoughts are full of pleasure, other less pleasant ones are dark and tumultuous, wreaking havoc on our inner landscape.

Cloud formations take on different forms depending on atmospheric conditions. Scientists identify these as cumulus, stratus, cirrus, and so on. Similarly, cognitive scientists have identified common styles of thinking that may contribute to unhelpful perspectives in thinking and therefore challenges with sleeping.

Below is a list of various common styles of thinking that often do us more harm than good. But the incredibly good news is that once we realize that the style of our thinking has taken on a particular tone, we can begin to untangle the stuck threads that are contributing to our suffering. Mindfulness can help us do just that. With mindfulness, we can become more aware of what is happening inside ourselves. When we begin to observe those processes without judgment, we develop a more accurate appraisal of ourselves and our situations. If this is done with compassion, we have a better chance of finding a wise and helpful response to our predicament, rather than continuing to be caught in the painful cycle that torments us in the middle of the night.

- **"Should" statements:** "Should" and "shouldn't" are common thought patterns that usually are not very helpful. They are attempts to compare ourselves to some idealized goal. Then, when we don't measure up, we're likely to feel inadequate and disappointed in ourselves. Telling yourself, *I should be able to fall asleep quickly and stay asleep all night* will likely lead to frustration and agitation because it is not actually reality.

- **Catastrophizing** is when you imagine the worst possible outcome from a situation. *If I don't get to sleep,* you tell yourself, *I won't be able to function at all and I'm going to lose my job.* Once this thought has taken hold, and you have blown up the problem into something huge, you experience the emotional impact as though the worst had already come to pass.

- **Labeling:** Attaching a negative label to a situation—or to yourself—can make a problem unsolvable by turning a temporary event into a permanent characteristic. *This is intolerable,* you might say, and then proceed to define yourself as "a hopeless insomniac"—which can easily lead to feelings of helplessness.

- **Fortune telling** is when you anticipate that things will always turn out badly and you are convinced that your predictions are accurate. *I am never going to be able to get a good night's sleep again,* you tell yourself. Ironically, when we really believe something to be true, our behavior may actually change unconsciously in ways that make it more likely that our negative predictions will actually come to be. A sad state of affairs for someone who was already suffering.

- **Disqualifying the positive:** It can be easy to discount positives in our lives and allow them to be eclipsed by our negative beliefs. We had some good nights of sleep while on vacation, but we discount that as a fluke and tell ourselves that it's not going to happen again.

- **Mood-congruent memory bias** occurs when your current mood influences which memories are called up. For instance, if you are feeling anxious, you will be more likely to remember other times in your life when you felt anxious, nervous, or worried, while at the same time ignoring those occasions when you have felt calm and at ease. As a result, you tend to overestimate how much of your life you have felt anxious, nervous, or worried, and you let those states define you. This can lead to other thought biases such as, *No treatment works for me,* and *I've tried everything already.*

- **Magnification and minimization** occur when we exaggerate our own screw-ups and inflate other people's achievements. If we stayed up too late reading Facebook, we call ourselves "a complete idiot," but if someone else does the same thing, we tell them, "Oh, you just got sucked into all those satire videos and cute kittens. No big deal." Holding different standards for ourselves than for others can make it difficult to see ourselves as anything but inferior to others.

- **Similarly, we are always comparing our insides to other people's outsides.** We don't have access to their thinking and perceiving, but we do to our own. People's outsides are usually a lot better than their insides because they are trying to put on a good face.

- **Personalization** is the thought pattern that says the bad things that happen in our life happen because we are flawed in some irreparable way. As a result, the positive things that happen to us are devalued—we attribute our success to luck, or being in the right place at the right time, while we think that bad things that happen to us are because we are by nature inferior. It may even seem that no matter what we do, there is some excuse as to why the things that happen to us are not as good as the same things that happen to others.

Guided Mindfulness with Acceptance Treatment for Insomnia (GMATI)

Guided Mindfulness with Acceptance Treatment for Insomnia (GMATI) takes behavioral treatment of insomnia in a different direction from what you may have been exposed to before. It seems to be more effective to teach people suffering from insomnia how to be more accepting of what they experience when having difficulty sleeping, rather than trying to directly change their sleep. This may seem strange, and yet this willingness to accept the experience of poor sleep can result in fewer struggles, less arousal, and, paradoxically, greater levels of calm, beneficial sleep. When you eventually learn to do this, like others already have, you will find that you are getting better and more sleep.

The key to this innovative, cutting-edge approach is the emphasis on changing your *relationship* with your sleep just as it is, by using mindfulness meditation. As you work into this new relationship with your sleep, you will begin to notice an improvement in the quality and then the quantity of your sleep. You will also find that you have more alertness and energy during waking hours, as well as better cognitive skills. All of this can usually be accomplished in a matter of weeks if you are diligent in working on it.

While cognitive behavioral therapy for insomnia (CBTI) directly addresses factors that interfere with sleep, GMATI, in contrast, is an indirect approach. As you practice these guided meditations during a portion of your daytime waking hours, you free yourself from the idea that it will directly improve your sleep. This last factor is really important, because if you meditate in order to accomplish better sleep, it can undermine its effectiveness. Rather, you will be instructed to do the meditations during the daytime and allow the effects to gradually carry over to work on your sleep for you at night. You do not have to do anything to make this carryover work. All you have to do is do the meditation during your waking hours, then allow its effects to indirectly improve your sleep (and usually your waking life as well). That is, you will not be directly trying to improve your sleep, but rather allowing the meditation to do this for you. All the people we have coached to do this have been able to do it, and have found that their sleep eventually improves both in quality and quantity.

So we invite you to try the GMATI approach to improving your sleep—and your life. The results can benefit you for the rest of your days.

CHAPTER 2

What's the Mind Got to Do With It?

Mindfulness: A Way of Allowing Sleep

Can GMATI, with its emphasis on mindfulness, help to allow sleep to occur naturally? What is mindfulness anyway? As a type of awareness cultivated through meditation, mindfulness has been around for over 2600 years. The form that we are most familiar with comes out of the teachings of the Buddha and has been passed down through Buddhist teachers for all these years. But it is also something that exists beyond "Buddhism," and there's no need to be a Buddhist to practice mindfulness meditation. Jon Kabat-Zinn, an internationally known proponent of mindfulness meditation and creator of the acclaimed mindfulness-based stress reduction program, describes it as "the awareness that arises when we pay attention, on purpose, in the present moment and nonjudgmentally." For the moment, let's think of mindfulness as cultivating a "relaxed awareness." It's about being attentive to where you are, just as you are, in the present moment, with a different, less reactive and more compassionate relationship to your thoughts, to the sensations in your body, in fact, to everything you may experience in your life. Even though mindfulness is mostly applied to experiences we have in our waking lives—and is, in fact, about being more awake and compassionately aware in our lives—healthy wakefulness can carry over and assist us in our sleep. Cultivating mindfulness throughout the day, as well as right before sleep, can help lessen the negative reactivity to not sleeping and increasing feelings of relaxation, thereby contributing to the conditions important for obtaining healthy slumber.

Most of us live the majority of our lives caught in our own habits and reactivity. Mindfulness is a pause from this that lets us expand our options and experiences simply by noticing what's actually happening—with compassion. Consider the notion of how you would explain water to a fish: take him out of swimming around in it for just one moment so that he can *see* what he's swimming around in. Mindfulness is our opportunity to be "taken out of" being automatically caught up in the stream of thoughts, feelings, and reactions and to just observe them instead. This shift from reactivity to compassionate observation has additional benefits, such as lessening the experience of pain itself, in both the mind and the body. For example, if feelings of anxiety and fear caused by worries and frustrations tumble forth from your mind as a result of insomnia, and you find them further keeping you from sleeping, your body may become tense as well. Mindfulness can help create a more balanced mental environment where that reactivity is reduced, making it more likely that the body can also relax and allow natural sleep to easily happen. This all occurs by noticing what's happening, not in some big story spread over time that we are telling ourselves, but in a simple, compassionate observation of this particular moment.

What Makes Up a Moment

Every moment that ever was or will be consists of an interplay between various components. Both Western cognitive-behavioral psychology and Eastern philosophies identify four major domains for human experience: (1) physical sensations, (2) thoughts, (3) emotions, and (4) behaviors. Each one is influenced by and influences all the others.

Imagine for a moment that you lie down and are trying to fall asleep. Now, add, for example, unwanted sensations of wakefulness: your body is energized and there is wakeful consciousness. Perhaps you also sense restlessness in some parts of your body, plus sensations of pressure or even of heat or cold. By themselves, these physical sensations are relatively neutral. They are only a "problem" because of the context in which they are occurring and your preference for things to be different. Now add thoughts: Your mind perceives the situation to be undesirable and perhaps even threatening. *If I don't get to sleep, I'm going to be completely dysfunctional tomorrow!* A complex of thoughts and emotions tumbles in to complicate your situation. *Why is this happening again? What's wrong with me? I can't stand this!* Emotions arise from there that could come in the form of frustration, agitation, grief, regret, sadness, anger, and so forth. Each of these emotions and thoughts carries an energetic charge, which in turn creates more tension in your body, resulting in even more restlessness. The behaviors that might go along with this scenario could be more tossing and turning, getting up and going to the kitchen, pacing, and so on. This downward spiral is not conducive to your sleeping.

Mindful Misgivings

As we have stated, mindfulness is focusing your awareness on something you are experiencing right now, but without evaluating it. Importantly, let's look at what mindfulness is *not.* Mindfulness is sometimes described as "mind-training" and "mental fitness," ideas which appeal to our cultural obsession with self-improvement. Too often, we ride the endless train of trying really hard to be anything other than what we already are. What we don't realize is that the very striving we are employing to become something else is, in itself, what is preventing us from ever feeling deeply happy and at ease. Worse, this striving to be different than we are at any given moment also has the effect of increasing tension in the mind and in the body, thereby activating the stress response. Too often, the end result is difficulty sleeping.

How does that stress show up? If your mind is continually getting the message that there is something wrong—like not being smart enough, or fast enough, or healthy enough, or never getting enough sleep—it interprets this message as a threat. As we saw in the last chapter, your brain's threat-detection system is well developed, but it's not very sophisticated. When we feel inadequate and are berating ourselves, our self-concept is threatened and so we attack the perceived problem—ourselves! Threat activates the fight, flight, or freeze reactions in the body. When this threat-defense system is turned in on us, fight becomes self-criticism, flight becomes self-isolation, and freeze becomes self-absorption (Neff & Germer, 2018). None of these is helpful when we are already suffering. Mindfulness is the first step to getting out of this.

Mindfulness is not a blissed-out, permanently calm state of mind. Being mindful, unfortunately, does not mean we're never going to get impatient or irritated again. "I meditate, I do yoga, I chant," says the meme circulating on Facebook, "and I still want to smack someone!" Mindfulness practice can help us calm our mind and react less impulsively, but no amount of meditation or mindfulness will stop us from being human. And being human means we get angry, we get agitated, we get impatient. We walk around, sometimes, with knots in our back or our jaw clenched. Or we feel sadness, or pangs of regret. We feel lots of things that we would rather not feel, that we wish would just go away and not bother us. Mindfulness is not about never experiencing those things.

Let's look again at the definition from Jon Kabat-Zinn. It is "the awareness that arises when we pay attention, on purpose, in the present moment and nonjudgmentally." Below, we further unpack this explanation of mindfulness.

A Further Explanation of Mindfulness

Awareness—of What?

Our species is called "Homo sapiens—the man-creature who knows." So just what is it that we "know"? If you are sitting while you read this, ask yourself if you can feel your rear end. Can you feel the sensations of pressure or warmth where your body is in contact with the chair? Most people answer yes. Now, the more interesting question: Were you aware of those sensations before you were asked the question? Most likely not. Typically, we're aware of our butts on a chair if there is pain or some other form of discomfort, but otherwise, those sensations are completely below our radar.

But when we bring our attention there, some sensation, or information, arises that can be known. This is what is meant by "awareness that arises."

Importantly, in addition to physical sensations, we can also be mindful of our thoughts and emotions. Rather than being caught up by them, we can simply be mindful of thoughts or emotions as if they are just things. For example, when we are absorbed thinking, *I am a hopeless insomniac,* we can instead view this statement as just words that we have in our mind. Or if we are anxious about our ability to sleep, we can tell ourselves, *I am experiencing anxiety about my sleep.*

On Purpose

You were just directed to bring your attention to your butt. Most of the time, we don't choose where we place our attention; it is captured by things. We see a beautiful sunset and our attention is drawn to it. We are right there, pulled in by the perception of beauty. We bang our shin on the open car door and we are right there, too, but this time with less pleasant sensations. Mostly, we are drawn by strong sensations, either pleasant or unpleasant. But all those moments of relatively neutral experiences usually seem to slip into the background and fade into a wash while our very interesting mind chatter takes over. We can, however, purposefully direct our attention to whatever we choose.

In the Present Moment

The present moment is the only moment there is to actually know anything. It is the only moment we have. In fact, it is only with our senses that we come to know anything about the present moment. Our senses are always happening in present time. For instance, we can't have a smell in the past. We can remember one, but while the mind is pretty masterful at recreating experiences from memory, if it's not actually happening now, it is only a thought, not an actual sensation. The smell of Grandma's apple pie baking in the oven is a direct olfactory experience while it is happening in the present moment. *Remembering* grandma's delicious apple pie baking is a memory. That memory may make your mouth water, but the nose is not actually experiencing the scent molecules of apple pie now. And so, in mindfulness, we are learning to become reacquainted with our own direct, sensory experiences in the present moment. They are what is happening *now.*

Typically, we are rarely here with our attention in the present moment. Our minds are actually somewhere else completely. Our minds are incredible time travelers. We cycle back and forth between the past and the future all the time. We journey to the past to rehash our experiences. We go over and over them, scouring every detail to look for new and important information. And we dream, plan, and fantasize about the future, rehearsing our role in it. We're constantly rehashing and rehearsing, past and future, but less often are we right here, right now.

This time-traveling function actually has a nifty name. Neuroscientists call it the "default mode network." If our mind is not absorbed in a task that we have intentionally set for it, it switches—or naturally defaults—to the default mode network. I picture it like a screen saver on my computer. It keeps the computer awake enough to be rallied back to action when I need it, but it's not necessarily doing anything on purpose; it's just sort of floating around being "on." It can also serve the function of daydreaming, problem solving, and so it's an important mode for the mind and so nothing to judge ourselves for experiencing. It's just not so helpful when we're talking about present-moment awareness. Have you ever had the experience of driving down the highway and looking up at an exit sign and remarking to yourself, *How did I get here?* If it's happened to you like it has to us, we have to ask, where *were* you during the time you were driving? Clearly your body was driving the car, but your mind was only partially there. It was wandering, telling stories of past or future. Fortunately, most of us are relatively operational and can still drive under these conditions. (This can also be a problem in our relationships when we're physically present, but are not really *there*.)

Another illustration of this comes from a wonderful cartoon from the *New Yorker* magazine in which a car is about to turn on to a long stretch of deserted highway. A huge road sign informs the driver "Your own tedious thoughts, next 200 miles." And isn't it like that in much of our lives?!

So we seem to make it to our destinations albeit accompanied by our own "tedious thoughts," but what about when we are trying to fall asleep at night? All these tedious thoughts can sure do a number on us, making it sometimes difficult to fall asleep. And as we saw in the last chapter, thoughts may be invisible and intangible, but they are not without energetic weight. They each have a vibrational charge that can be incredibly hard to bear. Like an electric outlet where some device is plugged in, these thoughts are constantly drawing energy and can definitely keep you awake.

Nonjudgmentally

This is both one of the trickiest aspects of mindfulness practice, and the main feature that makes a particular type of awareness "mindful." If what is being experienced in the present moment is not met with a lens of nonjudgment, it is not truly mindfulness.

The mind is constantly judging what it perceives. It says, *I like this,* and *I don't like that. This is good. That is bad.* Judgment seems to permeate every moment. And along with judgment come feelings. If what we are experiencing is judged as pleasant, we tend to try to hold on to it. However, if what we are perceiving is deemed unpleasant, we tend to resist and try to make it go away, which can lead to quite a lot of tension. And, as we saw before, if what we are experiencing is in the category of an emotionally neutral experience—we neither like it nor dislike it—the mind quickly jumps to something more interesting, and so we ignore the experience altogether.

In order to have a "nonjudgmental" awareness of something, we need to intentionally bring in other mind states or qualities. The two we find most helpful are *curiosity* and *kindness.* With curiosity, we are becoming deeply interested in what is here. (This is naturally easier to do if we are aware of something new to us, but harder to do with the ordinary or the familiar.) We are nonjudgmental when we suspend the automatic habit of dismissing an experience as already being known, and, instead, move in close, as if experiencing it for the first time. Adding a friendly or kind quality to the curiosity enables us to slow down a bit, move toward, and become more acquainted or intimate with the actual sensations of the moment, instead of just our preconceived notions of what we think it is, or should be.

Even if what we are noticing in our present-moment experience is a judgment of something, we don't need to judge that! Instead, applying curiosity, we can expand to a larger container of awareness by asking ourselves, *Hmm, what does this judgment actually feel like right now? What is happening in this judgment—in the body, in the mind? What is actually here right now to be known?* We can even experience the awareness of *judgment* with a nonjudgmental, kind, and curious attitude!

A Little Practice

We've spent quite a few pages defining what mindfulness is. But the only way to really know it is to actually experience it. And so to that end, take a few moments to try the raisin meditation as a way to begin to experience what mindfulness meditation is and how rich it can be with even a simple, familiar thing.

RAISIN MEDITATION

In almost any introductory mindfulness session with an individual, workshop, class, or lecture, we begin by doing something we all do every day, but this time, we do it mindfully. That thing is eating. And a simple thing to eat is a raisin. You don't have to love raisins and it's totally okay if you don't even like them (you probably don't like the suffering caused by insomnia either). So, go ahead, try this.

1. Start by holding two raisins in your palm. Focus the majority of your attention on the palm of your hand and just feel the raisins. You may even want to close your eyes to really concentrate your attention on the sensations in your hand. Feel their weight. How much space do they take up? Notice any thoughts or mental associations you have with raisins and try to just observe these

as thoughts and then let them move into the background of your awareness.

2. Next, open your eyes and start to really look at the raisins. You can even try to imagine that you were seeing raisins for the first time. You may have seen many raisins in your lifetime, but you have never seen *these* two.

3. Notice the colors, shapes, contours. You can start to "play" with them by using the fingers on your opposite hand to touch the ridges of the raisins and rolling them over in your hand.

4. Now, just pick one. Notice what happens in the choosing. Do you choose the one that is "prettier" or do you choose the "underdog"? (This is not to judge your choice, but to just be aware of all that goes into it.)

5. From here, really open your senses of sight and touch to get to know this raisin as intimately as possible.

6. Every once in a while, shift your attention from your hands and eyes to the rest of your body and notice how it is responding to this exploration.

7. Once you feel you have a good amount of familiarity with the sight and feel of the raisin, bring it up to your ear. Hold it between your thumb and forefinger and roll the raisin back and forth. Listen, does it make a sound?

8. Now, continuing to hold the raisin between your fingers, extend your arm and hold the raisin out in front of you. While keeping your eyes on it, start to bend your arm and *very* slowly bring it toward your mouth. Notice what is happening inside your mouth. Has the level of moisture in there changed? Your mind is perceiving a food item and is readying the body.

9. Bring the raisin to your lips and using the sensitivity of your lips, feel the sensations here. Continue to notice what's happening inside the mouth.

10. When and if you feel ready, place the raisin inside your mouth and let it rest on the tongue, but don't bite down. You are now introducing the sense of taste. Allow the taste of the intact raisin to come into the forefront of your attention. You are also feeling the sensations of it on your tongue. Notice how different the sense of touch is between fingers, lips, and tongue.

11. Experience how the tongue is a very curious muscle and is probably pushing the raisin up against the teeth.

12. Letting the tongue do its job of getting the raisin between the teeth, now bite down. Notice the experience of flavor and taste. And the strength of the jaw doing the chewing. And the changing shape of the raisin as it is crushed between the teeth. And also the ability of the body to draw

the pieces down the throat to continue the process of digesting.

13. Continue being present with the raisin until you can no longer distinguish it as separate from you.

14. When you are ready, open your awareness to the other raisin still resting in your hand and take your time following this same process to really get to know that one.

15. Now, think about how you were aware of a simple raisin in so many different ways by totally focusing on it in your immediate presence but without evaluating it.

What did you notice with eating the raisin in this way? Is this your usual way of eating raisins? What did you experience about the texture and taste? See what happens when you bring in curiosity to your experience. It opens you up to new possibilities and slows you down a bit. Now let's see if you can bring the same kind of curiosity and attentiveness into a more "typical" kind of meditation.

AWARENESS OF BREATH MEDITATION

In the same way that you just used your senses to savor two raisins, let's try doing the same thing with the breath.

1. Find a comfortable place to sit—either on a chair, or on the floor with cushions under your seat to raise the pelvis off the ground.

2. Let your back have a feeling of uplift, so that you can sit erect but not stiffly. As if you were a monarch sitting gracefully on your throne.

3. Allow your eyes to close or simply rest your gaze softly toward the floor. (We do this to minimize the amount of visual stimuli coming in, so we can turn our attention inwards.)

4. Let yourself feel the contact your body is making with the chair or cushion, letting your body know that you are right here now, in the present moment.

5. Notice what sensations may be present in the body as a whole and then gather your attention to focus on your breath.

6. Let your breath take the center stage of your awareness, as if you were using a camera lens and you heightened the focus on the breath. Other sensations are present, but they are simply in the background of your awareness.

7. Start to notice where you experience and feel the breath most easily. Maybe it's at your nostrils and you feel the passage of air coming in and out. Or perhaps it's at your chest and you feel the gentle rising and falling of your chest moving

from inhalation to exhalation. Maybe it's the subtle rhythmic expansion and softening of your belly.

8. It doesn't matter where; what matters is the clear and gentle awareness you bring to your breath, the one you are experiencing right now.

9. You can even place your hand over your belly or on your heart to make closer contact with your breath, and also as a reminder to bring a kind and curious attention both to your breath and to yourself.

10. When you notice that your mind has moved away from the breath and is engaged in thinking, no big deal. Just acknowledge to yourself that that has happened. Simply and silently say to yourself *thinking* or *thought* and then, with affection, as if you were leading a small child or a little puppy, escort your attention back to your breath—the one that is happening right now.

11. Do this for just a few minutes, even just three minutes, to simply allow yourself to touch the possibility of being with your breath, with yourself in this mindful, kind, and curious way.

Make Peace Not War

By now you may be getting a "taste" for what mindfulness is like and what it may have to offer. But remember, this is just the beginning. We have a lot we will offer you to help alleviate the struggle and suffering you're experiencing from insomnia. Later in the book, we will introduce you to other extremely beneficial practices that come from the "mindful self-compassion" program developed by doctors Kristen Neff and Christopher Germer. We will give you guidance and teachings that will help you develop both mindfulness and self-compassion. So we invite you to try the GMATI approach (which includes self-compassion) to improving your sleep—and your life. The results can benefit you for the rest of your days.

When you are training yourself to encounter life in this way, you are stopping a war. This is the exhausting war with life that we all wage by unconsciously grasping and resisting, trying to make life different than it is. This war is waged in our own minds and on our bodies, and it wreaks havoc on our well-being—including on our ability to sleep. Each time your mind creates catastrophic stories about the future because of how frustrated you are about not sleeping, you are inadvertently continuing this internal war. The brain interprets that train of thinking as a threat and reactivates the stress response.

Do Mindfulness and Self-Compassion Work?

You may still be wondering, "Will this really help me in the way it has helped many others?" The best way to answer that is to try it and see. At the end of the book, we'll look at what happened for the folks we told you about in the last chapter.

For now, think about it this way: To really rest, we need to feel safe and at peace. Humans are programmed that way: our cave-dwelling ancestors survived because they kept one eye open for saber-toothed tigers. But how can we feel safe and at peace? Mindfulness and self-compassion practices can give us that experience of peace because it's a peace that does not depend on an absence of difficulty. We can learn to encounter ourselves, encounter our lives, with acceptance and compassion and in so doing, bring about the conditions where we can let go into rest. That is our aim, and the rest of this book will help you do just that.

Research has shown that mindfulness and self-compassion practices are effective at treating stress-related conditions, as well as anxiety and depression (two conditions that are caused by and aggravate sleep disturbance). Mindfulness and self-compassion can quiet the war in our heads with a practice of peace. Peace becomes possible when we let go of our habits by which we force ourselves to be different from how we are in any particular moment. Instead, we can let go and allow ourselves to be exactly as we are. We can bring a sense of curiosity to observing what actually is—and then we are likely to see the moment dissolve and change on its own.

Clinical experience and results of initial scientific studies have demonstrated the effectiveness of carefully crafted mindfulness practices for improving sleep (Garland et al., 2015).

While the research on mindfulness for insomnia is accumulating, there is already an enormous body of scientific research demonstrating the power of mindfulness to help with many of the challenges that contribute to insomnia, including anxiety, depression, and pain. It's clear from our own clinical work that mindfulness practices can have a huge impact on the lives of people like you who are struggling with sleep.

In the previous chapter, we heard from a number of people who were struggling with insomnia. Each of them told us in their own way that after learning mindfulness and self-compassion techniques, their sleep, and their lives in general, were much improved.

Throughout this book, you will learn the same mindfulness and self-compassion practices that have already helped many people sleep better and find greater contentment in their lives. We will show you how practices taken from programs such as mindfulness-based stress reduction and mindful self-compassion, as well as other mindfulness and relaxation practices, can be used to alleviate the mental, emotional, and physical suffering caused by insomnia. You will learn to identify both internal and external factors that may be compromising sleep and how you can escape from them. Along with reading this book, you can access guided meditations that can be used: (1) throughout the day to train your mind and body to be less reactive to circumstances; (2) before going to bed to create new habits and wind down; and eventually (3) even in the middle of the night when you find yourself awake and need support.

With our guidance, you can do this!

CHAPTER 3

Sleep: Who Needs It?

It was late in the day when the young woman we'll call Sonja arrived at the university counseling center. She wore a winter hat pulled down over her forehead so that it almost covered her eyes, eyes that were puffy and red and more than a little vacant. She hunched her shoulders as she entered, then collapsed on the couch like she wanted to just be swallowed up by it. In a friendly but quiet manner, she talked about the incredible amount of anxiety she experienced. "I feel jumpy and jittery all the time," she said. "I can't concentrate in class and I feel paranoid, like nobody likes me." When asked about her sleep habits, Sonja answered, "What sleep? I haven't slept more than one or two hours in years." She went on to explain how she would study late at night and then play games on her iPad until the early hours of the morning. By then, she said, "my body feels like it will dissolve from exhaustion, but my mind is buzzing and racing and I toss and turn until about 4:00a.m., when I say 'forget it!' and then just go back to using my computer or iPad." She couldn't remember a time when she did sleep well. "My mom even says

42

that I was a bad sleeper as a baby and I figured over time that it just wasn't worth trying anymore. Yeah, I'm tired all the time, but why is sleep so important anyway?" We answered her question in the following way.

What Is "Normal" Sleep?

The answer to this is important for you, Sonja, and others who suffer from poor sleep. We have found during our treatment of people with insomnia that their misconceptions about sleep actually contribute to their distress. They experience some relief when they more factually and more fully understand sleep. Having such information helps lower their anxiety. We expect that this will also be true for you, so let's proceed with some accurate information about sleep.

Like most people, Sonja assumes that normal, ideal sleep is like that shown in figure 1, in which everyone supposedly needs about 7 1/2 hours of deep sleep without waking up. It turns out that this ideal is false. Let's look at what is really natural or normal.

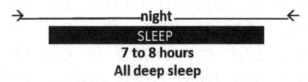

FIGURE 1. The modern Western world conception of ideal sleep.

First of all, nobody at any age sleeps continually through a typical night. Data from sleep-lab studies tell us that through the first four decades of life, a couple of awakenings is the norm. By the time you're in your forties and then onward, the number of awakenings increases as you age. When you reach your seventh decade of life, you may be averaging around nine awakenings. You may not be aware the next morning that you had woken up this many times, but it can contribute to your perception of a problem that you might then label as "insomnia," especially as you get older. However, it is not truly insomnia if you are aware of waking a few times at night—as long as you can fall back to sleep quickly (we will get to this later).

It's also important to understand that your sleep is not a unitary state. You alternate between REM and NREM sleep approximately every hour and a half throughout the sleep period. These two kinds of sleep are as different as they can be. NREM sleep is like a quiet bedroom, while REM sleep is like a family room with lots of activity. To make things even more interesting, there are three variations of NREM sleep, called N1, N2, and N3. It is difficult for you to easily awaken from N3; it is often considered deep sleep. If you do awaken during N3, you feel groggy and, importantly, you know you have been asleep. This is not true for N1, N2, and REM; they can be considered lighter sleep stages. If you awaken from any of these, you just cannot be sure that you were asleep unless if you recall that you were dreaming after awakening from REM.

During a normal night of sleep, you start out having more of the deep N3 sleep and only a little REM sleep and some N2 (N1 is a brief transitional state between wake and the rest of sleep), but the second half of the night contains little if any N3 and much more N2 and REM. Then, as age advances, you have less and less N3, especially later in the sleep period. Although this does not affect most people, it can contribute to the perception of initially sleeping well early in the sleep period, when deep N3 sleep is prevalent, but then not sleeping well during the second half of the sleep period, when the lighter types of sleep predominate. Thus you, like many others, may perceive insomnia to dominate the second half of the night, especially as you get older.

And then there is what we like to call the "sleep pause." Historical and scientific evidence reveals that it may be more natural for you to sleep in two distinct chunks, called first and second sleep, of three to four hours each, separated by one to two hours of wakefulness. See figure 2.

Prior to electric lighting, the sequence of first sleep then sleep pause then second sleep was understood as natural, normal sleep. The terms first sleep and second sleep were in common usage back then and were well understood. First sleep is dominated by deeper N3 sleep, while second sleep is primarily lighter NREM and REM sleeps. People back then did not consider the waking time between first sleep and second sleep as a problem or a waste of time; rather, it was a time of calm peace. They would use the sleep pause period for talking with bedfellows, praying, engaging in sex, reflecting on their waking lives, meditating on their dreams, and so forth.

It is now known that the sleep pause seems to have a physiological basis. The levels of the hormones melatonin and prolactin are higher during the sleep pause compared to during the sleep before and after it.

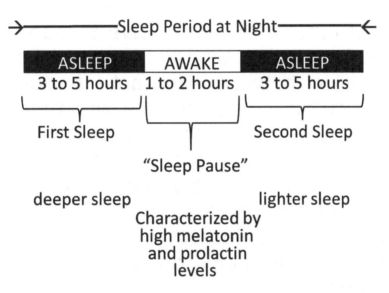

FIGURE 2. First sleep, second sleep, and "sleep pause."

With the advent of electric lighting, it became possible for people to "get things done" later in the evening and to wake up earlier in the morning. So rather than going to bed earlier, then falling asleep, then waking up for a couple of hours in this sleep pause restful state, then going back to sleep, you, like most people, probably expect that you should simply stay asleep for seven or eight hours straight, and that lying in bed awake in the middle of the sleep period is an annoying waste of time and a sign of insomnia. Yet modern scientific evidence shows that the biological tendency toward sleeping in two periods with a time of waking in between is still with us. Although it may have been possible to "sleep through the night" when you were younger, as you get older, your body may tend to sleep in two periods with a period of wakefulness in between.

This does not mean that you have to adopt the sleep pattern of first and second sleep with a period of being awake in between. In fact, in our society, it may be difficult for you to take the time necessary for sleep pause. The point here is that if you find yourself awake in the middle of the night, you can tell yourself that this is not abnormal, but merely your natural sleep pause manifesting itself, and that second sleep will follow. People with insomnia frequently tell us that realizing this helps reduce their anxiety about their insomnia.

How Much Sleep Do I Need?

"Okay," said Sojna, "but how much total sleep do I need per night?"

The answer is simple, yet challenging. You undoubtedly have heard that everyone needs close to eight hours of sleep per night. Surprise, surprise! This is not true. Yes, the majority of people require seven or eight hours to fulfill their biological sleep need, but others may need as little as five or six hours or as much as nine or ten hours. The difficulty comes with determining your individual sleep need. There is no way to determine this in a sleep lab or with biological tests.

The best you can do is this. If you are trying to sleep too many hours, you will tend to be awake in bed more. If you are not getting enough sleep, you may suffer from sleepiness and fatigue and their related problems during the day. So, adjust your sleep to be comfortably between these two. Of course, other things may keep you awake at night and other things may make you feel sleepy and fatigued during the day, both of which make this determination difficult. Nevertheless, it is important to try to have an awareness of your own sleep need.

Sonja then followed with a good question: "Why do we even need sleep?"

The answer to this question is important for those who suffer from sleep problems. We expect that this will be true for you, so let's continue with even more information about sleep.

Actually, the answer to the question, "Why do we need sleep?" has three components: What can sleep do for me? What happens during sleep to produce its benefits? Biologically, how is my sleep produced?

What does sleep do for us? And what happens during sleep to produce these benefits? You, like most people, would probably respond something like, "We need to sleep to restore, repair, and refresh the body, which has been worn down by hours of being awake." Surprisingly, scientists now believe that that's not the main reason we sleep. Sleep, it turns out, provides much more benefit for the mind than the body. See below.

The Benefits of Sleep

- Perhaps the most important mental benefit of sleep is for memory. When we sleep, our minds weed out the less important things we have recently learned or experienced. Right now, you can probably tell me what you had for dinner yesterday. After several days, this memory may be gone because it is no longer important to hold on to.

- On the other hand, when we sleep, important memories are strengthened and fitted into the organization of existing memories. If you just learned some new skill or fact that is valuable to your job, education, social life, or health (such as what you are reading right now), it will most likely stick around for months, years, perhaps even for the rest of your life. Your mind has trouble doing this when you are awake because it is too busy attending to the bombardment of sensory information, thoughts, and emotions of daily life.

Only during sleep, when it is largely free from all of this, can it attend to the memory tasks.

- Sleep also helps you think better while awake, enhances your ability to learn, makes you more creative, more attentive, and more flexible in your thinking, and enables you to make better decisions. Without adequate sleep, we tend to be more impulsive and more immature in our behaviors.

- Another important benefit of sleep is for your emotions. If you had a bad day and you are feeling really down, during sleep, your mind, especially through dreams, will endeavor to boost you up, and you wake up feeling better. In contrast, when your ego is overinflated, during sleep, again largely through dreams, you are cut back to a more realistic evaluation of yourself. Likewise, you can work through your emotional problems in your sleep. For example, Rosalind Cartwright and colleagues (1998) showed that people with a moderate amount of depressed mood at bedtime showed better mood after sleeping and dreaming because they were "working through" their problems. If there is nothing much for you to emotionally work on, you can even play in your dreams—and play is not a waste of time, but a healthy emotional activity.

- Another value of sleep is in problem solving and creativity. Historically there are many famous instances of this. For example, Robert Lewis

Stevenson woke up with the idea for his story "Dr. Jeckel and Mr. Hyde," Paul McCartney awakened with what became the tune for "Yesterday," and Elias Howe had the solution for his invention of the sewing machine after a night of sleep. Why? Again, our minds may be too cluttered up when we are awake, but free from that clutter, they can create and try out several solutions, then select the most favorable one. This more often occurs in your sleeping mind in less dramatic ways.

- During sleep, your less active brain has a chance to repair and restore itself, following the heavy use it gets when we are awake. Especially important is eliminating unwanted chemical buildup. This leaves the brain cleaner, healthier, and more efficient.

- The rest of your body does get some benefit from sleep. For example, you have more energy reserves to draw on after a night of sleep, and your immune system is given a bit of a boost by sleep.

But just what is the nature of sleep that enables us to obtain these benefits?

You might think, *Oh, I know this one! Sleep is when your brain shuts down.* Alas, a popular misconception! Your brain does greatly lower its overall activity during sleep, but it is still active. After all, we couldn't dream if our brains were shut off! But our brains do much more than just dream.

Instead of imagining your brain as "off" when asleep, think of sleep as a restructuring of the functions of your brain. It is well known that different areas of the brain have specific functions to perform. When you are awake, these different areas interact with one another in ways that allow you to function in your day-to-day life. However, when you are asleep, many of the interactions change. That is, your brain no longer needs to do all of the tasks it does when you are awake, so it can quiet down a bit. But even more importantly, it is functioning differently so that it can accomplish its sleep tasks, including dreaming. For example, when you are awake, the inputs and outputs of information in your hippocampus (which lies under the surface of the brain, from the middle to the back of each side) allow you to acquire new memories. When you are asleep, the inputs and outputs are changed such that your hippocampus can work on sorting out recently acquired memories instead.

You might also wonder how sleep is generated biologically.

There are two key systems that are involved in producing sleep: the sleep drive mechanism and the wake drive mechanism (the circadian clock).

Sleep Drive Mechanism

Like most people, you know that during the hours that you are awake, you accumulate a greater and greater need to sleep. Then, as you sleep, the need for sleep diminishes. This is called your sleep drive mechanism. Here is how it works.

Your three-pound brain makes up a small proportion (about 2%) of your body, but when you are awake, it consumes around 20% or more of your body's total energy. The consumption of this proportionally large amount of energy during the day creates an accumulation of byproducts that get cleaned out at night. Just as burning wood releases energy in the form of light and heat as the chemistry of the wood is changed, energy is released in your body when the structures of certain chemicals are changed. The burning of wood also creates byproducts such as smoke and ash. Likewise, byproducts remain, following the conversion of chemicals in your body to produce energy. Because the brain is so active when awake, it cannot keep up with getting rid of these byproducts (as well as other chemicals), and so they accumulate. When you sleep, there are physiological changes in the brain that enable it to clear away the accumulated chemicals. It is as if an hourglass fills up during the day and then at night is turned over so that the material flows in the opposite direction.

The bottom line here is that your current level of sleepiness depends on how much sleep you have gotten compared to how much you have been awake during the last couple of days to couple of weeks. Bear in mind this cycle of chemical buildup and cleaning out while we describe another factor.

Most of the brain is active when you are awake, but there are a few small portions deep in your brain that are less active. When you go to sleep, these areas become very active and take over control of your brain. These areas are responsible for producing sleep by temporarily restructuring how the brain functions. Without them, sleep would not occur.

Now, here is the interesting part. These areas of your brain, which are responsible for producing sleep, seem to be activated in proportion to the buildup of the chemical byproducts generated during waking energy consumption in the brain. The result of the activation of these areas is experienced as *sleepiness.* So while you are awake, your brain is consuming lots of energy, and the byproducts of that process are accumulating, resulting in ever-increasing levels of sleepiness. Then, as you sleep, your brain is able to gradually clear out these byproducts causing sleepiness to diminish (see figure 3). (There are other chemicals that also affect these sleep-drive areas, but they do not change the point we are making here.)

54

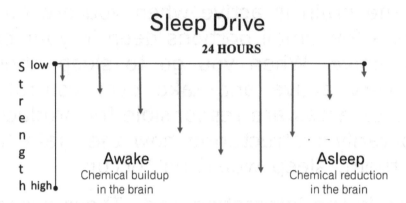

FIGURE 3. Sleep drive: Current level of sleepiness depends on the ratio of wake (+) and sleep (-) amounts during the last few days or weeks.

The Wake Drive Mechanism

While the sleep drive mechanism is facilitating sleepiness, another part of the brain opposes the sleep drive. This is the wake drive function of the circadian clock. The key point is that this clock, located deep in the brain, causes the opposite of sleepiness. That is, the output of your circadian clock opposes the action of the sleep drive mechanism and tries to keep you awake.

Your circadian clock is a single area deep in your brain that is about the size of the tip of your little finger. In human beings, the wake drive of the clock gets stronger as hours pass during daylight hours, but weaker with the passage of time in the dark (see figure 4).

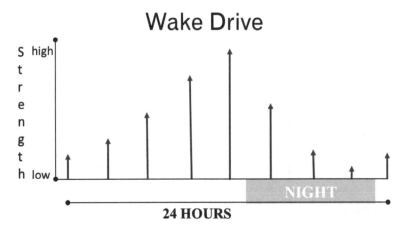

FIGURE 4. Wake drive produced by the circadian clock.

Your sleep drive and wake drive interact as shown by the solid wavy line in the middle of figure 5. During the day, even though sleepiness is increasing, you tend to stay awake because your circadian clock wake drive is also increasing and remains stronger than the sleep drive. At night, however, sleepiness from your sleep drive system is stronger than your wake drive from the clock, and so you tend to stay asleep. Morning comes and the relative strengths reverse again and you wake up and tend to stay awake until the next evening.

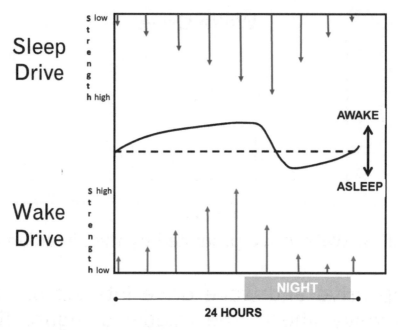

FIGURE 5. The interaction of the sleep drive system and the wake drive system.

Complexities of the Sleep/Wake Systems

Details of sleep drive and wake drive add several complexities that can be important in understanding your insomnia.

First, whenever you sleep—day or night—the process of the brain clearing out the excess chemical byproducts occurs. Thus, napping reduces the strength of the sleep drive in proportion to the length of the nap. Conversely, if you got insufficient sleep during the night, the level of the chemical byproducts may not be fully reduced, leaving a greater level of sleep drive still. Both of these can pose problems for people.

If the level of sleep drive is too low because of excess napping, then it is difficult for people to sleep well during the night. But if the level of sleep drive is insufficiently reduced at night, then daytime consequences result.

A second complexity in this sleep drive/wake drive interplay is that, left on its own, your circadian clock, as it does in most people, takes a few minutes longer than twenty-four hours to complete a cycle. This would cause it to gradually move its wake drive later with every passing day. Eventually, you would be very alert at night and find it difficult to sleep, while not being very alert during the day. But then the cycle would continue to move, until some time later it got back where it started. This cycle would continue to happen over and over again. This does not happen to most of us because every morning, when we awaken from darkness into light, the clock resets itself to keep it synchronized to our environmental day/night rhythm. Thus, you continue to be awake during the day and sleepy during the night. However, in some people, this daily resetting may fail, and they do suffer from swings of weeks of good sleep to weeks of poor sleep and back again. If this happens to you, you may think you have insomnia when it really is a problem with your circadian clock, which requires treatment not covered in this book.

Third, there are quirks in the setting of the circadian clock that affect the sleep period. In teenagers, everything moves later by an hour or two (or even more). Picture the wake drive arrows and the wavy line in the middle of figure 6 moving to the right by this amount. This means teens find it easy to stay up later at night but harder to get up in the morning. Careful studies have shown that this shift is a biological one, not primarily caused by simply desiring to stay up later at night. (Although evening activities, especially screen time, can exacerbate this shift.) The setting tends to gradually swing back in the other direction as teens age into their early twenties.

Later, as people get older, the opposite happens. Some people notice as they get into their forties that they get sleepier earlier in the evening and tend to wake up earlier in the morning than they did before. Picture the wake drive arrows and the wavy line in the middle of figure 6 moving to the left by an hour or two. By retirement age, for the majority of people, this becomes more common and more noticeable.

Both of these changes in the sleep period relative to the day/night cycle can contribute to the perception of insomnia. Teens may think they have sleep onset insomnia and older adults may think they have early awakening insomnia. (If extreme or intolerable, both can be alleviated with behavioral methods, but that is beyond the scope of this book.) Understanding that these changes are natural with age can alleviate the distress you may have of thinking that something has gone wrong with your sleep.

Fourth, during the middle of the afternoon, the strength of the wake drive produced by your circadian clock typically reduces for a bit of time, perhaps a half hour or so, as shown in middle of figure 6. This has been called the "midafternoon dip," and it results in midafternoon sleepiness. Like most people, you probably notice this at times but then experience a "second wind" as the circadian clock resumes its increasing level of alertness, as if this dip never happened.

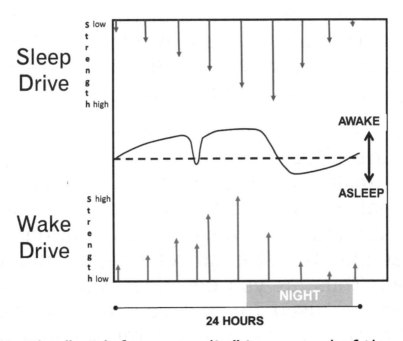

FIGURE 6. The "midafternoon dip" in arousal of the circadian clock and its effect on the level of wakefulness.

Often, people blame the midafternoon dip on lunch. However, it is not lunch that causes it, but this quirk in the circadian clock. Sometimes, people take a nap if their circumstances allow. Some cultures set aside this time for a siesta. Frequently, the dip is not strong enough to result in sleep, and other times, it may not be noticed at all.

Commonly, people who suffer from insomnia are told not to nap. The fear is that napping will reduce their sleep drive at night, thus making their insomnia worse. However, many sleep experts would say that a brief nap of twenty or thirty minutes is permissible for most everyone without greatly affecting subsequent nighttime sleep, even people with insomnia, and can be beneficial, because mental alertness, efficiency, and mood are usually enhanced by naps. Furthermore, a midafternoon nap can be considered biologically natural because the circadian clock encourages it.

Fifth, from middle age on, the resultant interaction between the sleep drive and wake drive (the wavy line in the middle of figure 6) flattens a bit for several reasons that are beyond the scope of this book. That is, the strength of wakefulness during the day diminishes plus the strength of sleep at night is a bit diminished. Thus, as you get older, you may not sleep as well as you used to, and you may be less awake during the day. These are natural changes with age that can contribute to your perception of insomnia.

Up to this point, we have emphasized the biological regulation of sleep. These are the sleep drive mechanisms in the brain that mechanically interact with the wake drive area in the brain. But, of course, there is more to the story. We call it the "right box" (see figure 7).

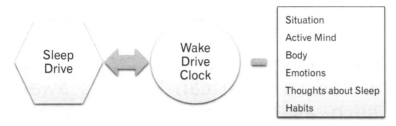

FIGURE 7. Including the "right box" with brain mechanisms that influence sleep.

Has this ever happened to you? You have been awake all day. You are sleepy. You go to bed at your usual time, expecting to soon fall asleep. But your neighbors are having a loud party that keeps you awake. This is an example of something in your situation that hinders the natural biological mechanisms for sleep. Other things might include traffic noise, sound from a TV, people talking, thunder, and so forth. These situational factors affect all of us at some point when we are trying to sleep.

One of the most common things that people with insomnia complain about is that their mind is so active that they cannot sleep. Sound familiar? Often at night, your mind might be dwelling on problems and concerns or future plans or reviewing the prior day or other past events. But it can also be full of a part of a song that continually recycles. Whatever the content, there seems to be no control over it—and the result is a disruption in your sleep!

Then there are the things in our bodies that can inhibit sleep. Pain is an example. But so are indigestion, allergies, tinnitus, cramps, fever, side effects of drugs, and so on.

Our emotions can likewise hinder sleep. Fears, anger, melancholy, and so forth can keep us awake. Positive emotions such as excitement, joy, amusement, and elation can also interfere with sleep.

Then there is the fact that people with insomnia often dwell on their sleep and what they wrongly assume it should be like. Such thoughts can also hamper sleep.

And finally, people suffering from insomnia often adopt habits that counter sleep. One example is spending extra time in bed in order to make up for the sleep they are having trouble getting. Usually, the result is more time awake in bed. Too often, this unconsciously causes them to associate bed with being awake rather than sleeping, thus contributing to their insomnia.

For a few people, the insomnia they experience may be primarily due to poor sleep drive, either inherited or the result of a brain injury. Or in some people, insomnia is primarily because of problems with their circadian clock/wake drive. But by far the most common contributors to insomnia are simply the factors in the "right box," which exacerbate the insomnia principally caused by sleep drive or wake drive problems.

The things just presented may seem pretty dismal when it comes to your sleep, but hang on. There is a lot you can do, more than you might think, to make your sleep better. In particular, the rest of this book will show you what you can do, especially about these "right box" factors that contribute to your insomnia.

PART 2

The Practicals of Practice

CHAPTER 4

GMATI—Week 1

Introduction to Working with GMATI

We've looked at mindfulness and we've looked at sleep. Now we're going to pull it all together for you. You may be feeling excited, skeptical, and probably still exhausted. This is all okay. Come to this exactly as you are.

We want to get you started on the first guided mindfulness meditation of the Guided Mindfulness with Acceptance Treatment for Insomnia (GMATI) program. Mindfulness is the heart and start of the program. If you've done meditation before, you'll recognize that for the most part, this first practice is a standard guided meditation. But it also includes important elements that lay the groundwork for the weeks to come.

We're going to be with you each day, and as we go along, you'll be deepening your experience of mindfulness as well as your ability to sleep more fully. Each week contains a specific theme and each day contains a specific practice skill. Each day, you will read about a teaching that you can use as a touchpoint for supporting and deepening your meditation practice. This first week and the next one also include some basic tips for getting started in your meditation practice.

We suggest journaling at the end of each daily section. Use it to note what you are becoming aware of in your practice as well as to track your practice. The journaling is not there to judge you or be something you need to beat yourself up over. Nonjudgmentally noticing what is arising in our bodies, mind, and mood is a powerful tool for self-understanding and helps in developing inner wisdom as well as self-compassion. Additionally, tracking what you are actually experiencing and doing in your practice is a powerful tool in helping you develop new habits.

Each week before you get started, we recommend that you first read through the new meditation to familiarize yourself with it. But reading a meditation is not the same thing as practicing it. It's essential that the GMATI guided meditation be done daily. You will find each meditation in a guided recording on the New Harbinger website (http://www.newharbinger.com/42587). Feel free to download each week's meditation so that you can listen any time you like during the day, one time per day during the week. This first meditation takes only about fifteen minutes to complete. We'll also be suggesting other meditations (many of which also include guided recordings) that you can use in addition to the GMATI meditation.

GMATI Week 1

The theme for this week is to develop mindful awareness of your sleep. You'll also be laying a foundation for mindfulness as a lifelong support for dealing with insomnia, as well as for relating to yourself throughout your life.

The main practice this week will be the GMATI-1 meditation. You'll also be learning how to incorporate mindfulness in everyday activities, and how to use the breath and body sensations as an anchor for your attention.

Your mindfulness practice should to be done during the day. You may be wondering what doing a mindfulness meditation during the day has to do with helping you sleep at night. Hang with us. We promise that as you get further along, you'll see how the focus becomes more and more on sleep. But for now, it's really important that you practice meditation once per day and only during the day. Don't try to do it at night as a trick for getting you to sleep. The paradox that exists in this whole thing is that the more you try to make sleep happen, the more tension is created, and the more elusive sleep is. So by doing the meditation during the day, you will not directly be trying to improve your sleep. The mindfulness meditation does this for you indirectly. All you need to do is do the meditation.

Meditation Tips for Week 1

As you progress through this week, we are going to offer daily meditation tips to help you get the most out of your meditation practice. Rather than just rushing into the daily practices to get them out of the way, consider being thoughtful about them and finding ways to change or adjust what you are doing to get the most out of them. These meditation tips are not admonishments or *musts,* but just friendly reminders that can help you.

As we mentioned in chapter 1, when you try to control your sleep and the discomforts of insomnia, you actually make things worse. The struggle for sleep worsens insomnia. Thinking about past nights of difficult sleep or about what will happen in the future because of another night of poor sleep only makes things worse. Making judgments about how things are "good" or "bad" also contributes to your insomnia. Additionally, all these thoughts and subsequent emotions use up a lot of energy, which makes you feel even more tired than if you were simply awake without the struggle. Attempting to excessively control sleep is like struggling with quicksand: it costs you a lot of energy and makes everything worse.

But there is a way out. In this week's meditation, and all the meditations that follow, you will be learning to just *accept* your sleep rather than trying to change it. This will actually indirectly improve the quality and quantity of your sleep and save energy for the next day.

You may be saying to yourself, "All right! So let's get this show on the road!" But remember, you are learning a new skill and it will take a few weeks to get there. We know it's incredibly hard to have patience when you're exhausted and just want relief. It's probably the hardest thing. What might help is to remember that patience is another way of being kind to yourself. And self-kindness or self-compassion is an essential part of mindfulness.

Okay, let's get started by reading through the first GMATI meditation!

GUIDED MEDITATION FOR GMATI-1

When you are in a comfortable sitting position, connect with an *intention* that will support your practice. It could be something like "*I'm taking this time to be with myself and allow myself and this moment to be exactly as they are.*" You don't need a three-page vow, even a word or two will do. Some I like to use are *"Be kind," "Be curious," "Be at ease," and "Be here now."*

And then just welcome yourself into the present moment. There is nothing right now that you need to be or to do. For these few moments, let go of the need for things to be different from how they are right now, and instead allow yourself to simply be aware. Let yourself be exactly as you are, and let your life be exactly as you find it. You don't need to be relaxed or happy. There is nothing that needs to be fixed. This is simply a time for you to befriend yourself, just as you are.

Begin to notice all the places that your body is in contact with something solid. It could be the chair under your seat, the ground against your legs or feet, your hands resting in your lap. Allow yourself to feel these sensations of contact and enable the body to know that in this very moment it is being held and supported, and that it is safe. Gravity is holding you in place. You don't need to work too hard to be sitting here, so you can let the weight of your body be totally supported by whatever you are resting on. You can let go of any unnecessary tension or holding on.

In addition to the sensations of contact with solid surfaces, see if you can also feel how your body is in contact with space. Maybe you notice the passage of air against your skin, or the feeling of temperature. Feel where you end and the space around you begins.

Now, as you feel into this, you may notice that your body is actually in a very dynamic relationship to space, because in this very moment, it is breathing.

So allow yourself to feel the sensations of breath in the body. How the air comes in on the in-breath and causes the body to expand, and then how the body gives up and releases the air on the out-breath, causing the body to soften and recede back. You may notice the sensations of breath at the nostrils, or in the chest, the belly, or some combination of these places. Wherever you feel it most vividly, allow this region of the body to become like a home base for your attention. It's like your attention is an adjustable lens, featuring the sensations of breath. For now, let sounds, thoughts, emotions, and other body sensations be in the background of your attention.

Breathe in and know that you are breathing in. Breathe out and know that you are breathing out. There is no need to change or control the breath in any way. Simply let the natural rhythm of your own breath be as it is, and just notice it moment to moment.

When you notice that your mind has wandered away from being aware of the sensations of breath, this is not a problem. In fact, you can even gently congratulate yourself for being aware that this has happened. Simply acknowledge wherever the mind has gone. You may even want to make a mental note and call the experience "thinking." And then, kindly and deliberately, escort your mind back to being aware of breathing.

As best you can, bring a quality of kindness and compassion to your awareness. Just breathing in, breathing out, moment to moment.

This same attitude of gentle allowing and acceptance can be brought to your entire experience of this moment. There is nothing to be fixed, no particular state to be achieved. Simply allow your experience to be your experience, with no need to be other than what it is.

Now, expand your attention around your breath and begin to notice other sensations in the entire body. Notice the changing nature of physical sensations, how they come and go. The itching, tingling, aching sensations. The areas of pressure or the areas where there is little or no sensation. So many sensations in the body. Be mindfully aware of how they arise and then pass.

Now, move your attention from the sensations in the body and place it in your ears, and in your sense of hearing, becoming aware of any sounds that are present right now. Sounds from your own body, sounds in the room where you are, sounds even outside the room. See if you can just allow yourself to receive the sounds.

Often there is a tendency in hearing to go searching for sounds and label them or analyze them, judging and evaluating them as good or bad, liked or disliked. Instead, simply receive the sounds meeting your ears. Just the raw experience of hearing. You can become aware of tone, pitch, sharpness, dullness, rhythm, and so on. But just be present in the hearing. Notice how the sounds come and then go. How they are constantly flowing and changing.

Now, let the awareness of sounds recede into the background of your attention, and bring your awareness to the activity of thinking. To the ability of the mind to create thoughts. Thoughts come in the form of images or narration. And yet, they too come and go. Thoughts themselves, like sounds and body sensations, are constantly changing.

Notice the mind developing plans, going over memories. The mind is so busy thinking about this, thinking about that, reacting, hoping, dreaming, remembering. But by being aware of the activity of thinking, you can begin to know that they are just thoughts. You can observe them like clouds moving through a vast sky, just making room for the thoughts to be as they are, and observing them as they come and go.

Thoughts may also take on an emotional charge. With your mindfulness practice, you can make room for those, too, allowing any tension, anxiety, boredom, or irritation to simply exist, just letting them be there as they are. Perhaps becoming aware of how they feel inside the body and observing how emotions too change from moment to moment—sometimes growing stronger, sometimes growing weaker, and sometimes lingering on for a while. For these few moments, it does not matter; just let them be.

The purpose of this practice is not to make you feel better. It is to help you get better at feeling, and at *allowing* whatever feelings are part of this moment.

Now, let the thoughts move into the background of your attention and widen your awareness as broadly as you like. You can imagine that your attention is like a wide-angle lens, taking in the phenomena that make up the full scope of the moment, making room for whatever is most predominant in your experience of this moment. Perhaps it is a sound, or a thought, or a body sensation. Just observe and experience each as it is arising and passing.

The object of your attention is the *present moment itself.* Mindfully observing the constantly changing nature of life.

If at any time you feel lost or overwhelmed by all that is arising, you can always come back to the breath, using the breath as an anchor for the attention. And then, when you are ready, open up the lens of your awareness once again. Open to whatever is arising. Just resting in presence itself.

Now, gather your attention back in to the breath once again. Return to having the breath in the foreground of your awareness—being mindful of the inhalation and the exhalation, moment to moment.

In these last few moments, try allowing yourself to feel some gratitude for having made the effort to engage in this practice for the sake of your health and well-being. Take time to simply be present with your experience as it is, without the need to make it any different. Without the need to do anything except to be aware, and to rest in simple presence.

Now, gently allow the eyes to open and take in the room that you are sitting in. Then bring some small stretching movements into your body before returning to the activities of your day. As you do, be aware that this feeling of presence, of focus, that we have just experienced is as close as the next moment—as close as the next breath.

Day 1: Establishing a Practice

Today, we're going to work on finding an easy, comfortable position to support the development of your mindful awareness and you're going to experience your first GMATI meditation.

When first starting meditation, it's worth taking some time to find a sitting position that works for you. One that is comfortable but also steady, with your back straight but not rigid. You don't need to imitate pictures of the Buddha or yogis. Find what works best for you. Here are a few additional suggestions:

- It's fine to use a chair—there's nothing special about sitting on the floor, although some people find it more comfortable. If you use a chair, choose one that has a straight back and allows your feet to be flat on the floor with your legs uncrossed. It is best, if you can, to sit well away from the back of the chair so that your spine is self-supporting. If you need to, you can place a pillow behind you to support your lumbar area.

- Many people find a bench the ideal way to get the right posture—you can experiment with adding cushions or a folded blanket to get the height just right for you.

- You can choose to sit on a cushion cross-legged on the floor, or on a stool or cushions with your knees in a kneeling position.

  - If you choose to sit cross-legged, find some cushions that raise your bottom three to six inches off the floor. Make sure your pelvis is slightly tilted forward and your knees are in contact with the floor. If they don't reach, you can place some small pillows or rolled towels beneath them. When you sit with your knees lower than your hips, your lower back will have a gentle inward curve and your spine will be self-supporting. Rest your hands in your lap or on your thighs. Experiment with these different ways of using cushions and supports to find a posture where you feel comfortable and firmly supported.

- You can also choose to sit in a kneeling position with the cushions under your seat. This enables your pelvis to be even higher off the ground and for the hips to avoid any external rotation. Support the comfort of your knees by placing a small blanket under them.

However you sit, feeling safe and grounded is an important step at the outset of any meditation. It helps you establish yourself in the present moment and provides the experience of stability. Also, during your meditation, you may have become very relaxed, and it's easy to start to feel a little slouched and unbalanced. Grounding yourself basically just means getting a renewed sense of your body in contact with the earth in the present moment. Your body is held and supported by the ground; it's the chair and cushion that is holding you.

Let your hands just rest on your knees or in your lap. Allow the shoulders to soften. You can even imagine sitting as if your shoulder blades were melting down your back. Sometimes this can cause the chin to poke forward, and if you find that's true for you, just soften your chin and allow for a feeling of opening at the back of the neck.

SETTING YOUR INTENTION

- "Setting your intention" means focusing and devoting yourself to the guided meditation you are about to experience. This is a very easy thing to do. As mentioned above, you can simply come up with a statement that helps you to feel dedicated to your guided meditation experience. Then, repeat that statement to yourself, either in your mind or softly out loud, just before you begin to meditate. You can start by connecting with what it is that is driving you to seek a meditation practice, such as by saying to yourself: "I desire to accept myself as I am and I am committed to being with myself in a kind and friendly way for the next twenty minutes." Or, "It is my time to meditate. Nothing more. I will let go of everything else."

- Your positive intention statement should be something meaningful to you alone. Avoid making it too long. A few carefully chosen words may be all you need.

- Notice how this works for you. Your intention may be something you decide once and for all. Or it may be something that is unique to how you are today. By taking a few moments to notice how you are before you start your practice, you can see what it is you need to support you.

  While it's true that the position of the body does not totally determine whether something is or is not a "meditation," the posture the body is in does indeed influence how at ease and alert you feel. Try it out for yourself:

- First, try tensing your body into a stiff, militarylike rigidity. See how this feels for a few moments. What do you notice happening to how the breath is flowing and the level of ease the mind feels?

- Now, try slouching in your chair, letting your head flop and your shoulders round forward. How alert and aware do you feel now?

- Okay, now try to find something in between these two postures and see how that feels. Imagine that you are a monarch sitting regally on your throne. You have an upright posture that embodies a relaxed dignity.

  If it's comfortable for you, allow the eyes to close or simply let your gaze rest down toward the floor and be relaxed and unfocused. See how this feels.

Now it's time to practice with the GMATI-1 meditation! Just before you do, start to consider what personal intentions you might have for doing this practice. You can go ahead and reread the above tip called "Setting Your Intention" to get some ideas, and then listen to the guided recording at the website for this book: ht tp://www.newharbinger.com/42587.

***

Congratulations! You've just begun a powerful practice that will help you with your sleep and with every aspect of your life!

Now one more thing. We recommend that you keep a journaling diary. This will indicate how long you meditated and start tracking what is happening for you with your practice. Remembering that nonjudgment is at the heart of mindfulness, what did you notice:

- In your body?

- In your mind?

- And in your mood?

Day 2: Cornerstone Attitudes

Welcome back! Today, before again meditating with the GMATI-1 recording, let's talk about some of the attitudes that are foundational in mindfulness practice. We look at them like cornerstones in a foundation for construction of a new building. The cornerstones align the foundation so that it will be true, solid, and stable. This is likewise true for constructing a mindfulness practice. So here they are:

Show Up

Show up to practice every day. This does require dedication and commitment. But this "stone" is also about *how* you show up. It's about being present with yourself and with whatever is showing up in the present moment—the good, the bad, the ugly. All of it. You only have this moment to live. And this moment will never be exactly like this again. Every moment is here—and then gone.

Listen Well

This "stone" is about our tendency to either hyperfocus or numb out to our own interiority. We hyperfocus by ruminating on our thoughts and our stories about ourselves. And so often, those thoughts and stories are biased and judgmental (just like the thought biases we explored in chapter 2). Our thoughts and feelings get magnified or minimized depending on our circumstances. Many of us are so out of touch with what's happening inside us that we're a little like sheepdogs—they have so much fur that when they're caught out in the rain, they have to get soaked to the bone in order to even know that they're wet. By attending to our own moment-to-moment experience as if we were deeply and empathically listening to a beloved friend, we begin to cultivate a good friendship with ourselves.

Speak the Truth Without Judgment or Criticism

This one is about developing a compassionate honesty with whatever is happening. As we've mentioned before, it's so easy to mistakenly think that mindfulness is about creating some kind of blissful or relaxed feelings. So we need to remember that it's about moment-to-moment nonjudgmental awareness with whatever is happening, whether it feels pleasant, unpleasant, or totally neutral. When you do your reflection at the end of your practice, try speaking what is true for you without judging or criticizing yourself or your experience in meditation.

Meditation Tip—Do the Meditation Daily

Be sure to do your guided meditations once per day at least six days per week. This is particularly important for two reasons:

1. The guidance is really important not only for learning the practice, but also for practicing the *attitudes* that are helpful in mindfulness. The language used in the guidance is very intentional and is there to help frame your mind to support the development of mindful awareness. We've noticed that some people have a tendency to overanalyze guided meditations when they first listen. Instead, endeavor to just "go with the flow." The more you do your meditations, the more you will become accustomed to meditating. You'll become familiar with the instructions and you'll start to feel acquainted with the speaker. We will be together for the next few weeks (and perhaps a lot longer), so it's important to become familiar with each other.

2. The positive effects of guided meditations accumulate. So even though you will experience benefits from your guided meditations initially, as

you continue to meditate, the benefits you experience will become increasingly deeper.

Let Go of the Attachment to Outcome

This can seem very frustrating because of course you are attached to an outcome, and that outcome is more and better sleep. But let's look at what actually happens when we're attached to sleeping a particular way. Usually this striving causes more tension, and then sleep is even more elusive. Then resistance to the moment sets in, and this leads to frustration, grief, and more suffering. So instead of thinking that doing the meditations will make you sleep better, think of it as a practice that removes the obstacles to suffering around issues with sleep. These obstacles are tension-filled resistance to what is happening in the present moment.

The attitudes that help us lay these cornerstones are:

Be Kind
This means your meditation needs to be infused with kindness. Having an affectionate attention toward yourself and whatever you are experiencing allows you to meet the moment with less struggle.

Be Curious
This one is really important! It is said that it is impossible to not be mindful if you are curious. And you can be curious about anything. Whatever is

happening in your meditation practice, whether it be boredom, agitation, even nothing, try bringing a childlike curiosity to the experience. You might even ask yourself questions like, "What does this boredom actually feel like? How is it showing up for me right now? What is happening in my body and mind that tells me that this experience is 'boredom'?"

Be at Ease
As with kindness, it's important to support your meditation practice with a spirit of physical and mental ease. When you find yourself striving or resisting, you need to relax and then investigate with curiosity your experience of striving or resisting.

Be Here Now
Easier said than done. Yet the only moment we ever have to cultivate mindfulness is the one that is happening right now.

Okay, with these things in mind, now it's time to meditate using the GMATI-1 recording.

***

When you're finished doing the meditation, don't forget to acknowledge all the effort you are taking to develop this practice and how you are being a good friend to yourself by doing so. Then, take a few minutes to add to your journal. Remembering that nonjudgment is at the heart of mindfulness, what did you notice:

- In your body?

- In your mind?

- And in your mood?

Day 3: The Usual Suspects

Now that you've had a couple of days of practicing the GMATI-1 meditation, we're going to take a look at some of the most usual reactions or observations people have when they begin meditating. By normalizing these experiences, you can shift from the tendency to label these as *problems* to "This is just what is happening." This is a powerful way to learn to accept yourself and whatever is happening in the present moment.

Take a moment now to just pause and ask yourself—what have you discovered when you've been doing this meditation? There are endless possibilities. Here are a few of the most common themes that come up, and also how you might work with them.

Meditation Tip—Make a Space for Meditation

A great way to enhance your guided meditation is to create a quiet, undisturbed atmosphere where you intend to practice it. Dim the lights and do what you can to ensure privacy. This may not always possible for you to do. If it is not, then you can just be mindful of whatever is happening—kids coming in, pets crawling onto your lap, and so on. These things are not "distractions," but just other things that may be happening at any given moment and that can then be simply noticed with compassion.

"My mind won't stay still."

This is an incredibly common observation with all meditation practices. In fact, it happens to everyone to varying degrees. It's not just you. Many people single themselves out by saying "*my unique* mind," as if their minds are of a very special jumpy, wandering variety. The fact is that all minds think. That's simply what they do. In many meditation teaching circles, the mind is likened to a monkey swinging from tree to tree, just as the thoughts jump from one thing to another. This is not a problem during meditation. In fact, even saying to yourself during a meditation, "Oh, that's thinking, no problem," or "Thinking is happening, no problem," can be a way of retraining your expectation regarding monkey mind.

Another image that is helpful to use when working with a busy mind is to imagine that the mind is like a scampery little puppy. Puppies, soft, cute, and fuzzy, do not sit still for very long. They are curious and are prone to wandering. When you are training a puppy to sit, you have to repeat the instruction over and over again and guide it back into sitting when it wanders off. Puppy training requires kindness and patience. So too with the mind in meditation.

"I feel bored, anxious, jumpy."

This is also extremely common, and it also is not a problem. These are all perfectly human experiences and do not imply that something is amiss. It doesn't take long while we are sitting in meditation to start thinking about all the other things we "should be doing." Restlessness can arise as the body "unwinds." When we sit to meditate, it's as if we've spent the day cooped up on a rocking boat. Once we come to shore, it feels as if our body is still moving and rocking. It takes time for the body to settle down and feel at rest. Meditating is like shifting gears in a car—you shift into neutral and the engine takes a while to slow down and come to idle. Such feelings are impermanent experiences, which, if just observed and acknowledged, will eventually change into something else.

"I feel sleepy and even a little spacey," or "I feel so relaxed."

These are not problems, either. But remember that although relaxation is pleasant, it is not actually the goal. When the mind is getting redirected out of its constant oscillation between past and future, the rest of the body may often start to slow down. We can also use this as an opportunity to allow the feelings of exhaustion and sleepiness when we are fed up with feeling them and still not able to sleep. In the same way that you might work with anxiety, restlessness, or boredom, just feel what sensations in the body accompany the feelings of fatigue. Notice them and see if you can just let them be.

"I notice a lot of pain in my body. I can feel all the aches and pains I didn't even know were there."

Being aware of any kind of pain, physical or emotional, can be extremely difficult. So it's really important to be kind to yourself. And the practice for how to work with it is exactly like all the other things we've listed. First, start by acknowledging the pain. Then I have a couple of options about how to be with it. Just like other things, you could bring an attitude of curiosity to the pain. Notice whether it is achy, throbbing, stabbing, prickly, and so on. You can imagine sending breath into this area, as if you could breathe right into or around the painful sensation. At any time, if the pain feels too strong to pay attention to, you can always bring your attention back to your breath to stabilize your attention and bring yourself some compassion.

"Am I doing this right?" or "This isn't working."

These can also be extremely common thoughts that people experience when they are new to meditation.

It's normal to feel unsure about something you are not used to doing, especially when you are really wanting something to happen in a particular way or if you're attached to a specific outcome. Here is an opportunity to remember that mindfulness practice is not about achieving any particular state. There is no "good meditation" or "bad meditation." It is about learning to be with ourselves exactly as we are, no matter what is happening.

Whenever you hear yourself thinking that it's not "working," ask yourself what you were expecting to happen. Then you can acknowledge the very human tendency to be goal focused. You could even smile at yourself and say, "Aha! Human again!" and then return to the practice of being nonjudgmentally aware of whatever is happening, knowing that that is simply how it is, and that, like all things, it will come and go. Just being with the unfolding of that moment too. This kind of awareness is a skill to cultivate in and of itself, and it also requires some patience, a kind spirit, and maybe a little humor. Patience, kindness, and humor are all attitudes you can experiment bringing to yourself in your meditation practice and in your life.

Okay, time to use to the GMATI-1 meditation recording again.

***

Once you finish, take out your journal and jot down some things that you noticed happening for you. Remembering that nonjudgment is at the heart of mindfulness, what did you notice:

- In your body?

- In your mind?

- And in your mood?

Day 4: Everyday Mindfulness

You've made it halfway through the week. Congratulations! There is tremendous value in being seamlessly engaged in mindful awareness throughout our lives. However, you may be finding that developing a daily meditation practice can sometimes feel a bit daunting. Carving out the time to decondition the constant impulse to be "doing something" can feel like a radical act. If that's true for you, you are not alone. It is really quite something that our lives are so full that we can't find ten or twenty minutes to spend with ourselves to cultivate mindfulness. Too often we feel like we need to be "doing something," so we fill our days being active with one thing or another. Yet we tell ourselves that taking time to meditate does not count as something we've "accomplished." So today, we'll look at how to weave mindful awareness into your everyday activities. When we have concrete and accessible ways to weave mindfulness into our lives, we can make different choices about how we savor the moment or release the things that are stealing our moments.

Sometimes, hearing about how others worked with something can be really helpful. So let us introduce you to a client, Chris, who asked (maybe like you're wondering), "How the heck am I going to find time to practice meditation when I already feel so maxed out and exhausted!?"

To answer that, he was encouraged to find something that he already did every day, in order to cultivate mindfulness by making it a "meditation." He spoke about how every morning, before his wife and three boys get out of bed, he goes down to the kitchen to make the coffee. It is a ritual for him. "I love how quiet it is at that time. And, I love my coffee." With help, he came up with a plan that the moment he entered the kitchen he would bring his attention into the sensory experiences of making and drinking coffee. He would allow his ears to hear the opening of the box of filters and his mind to register the sensations in his muscles while he scooped out the beans. He would allow his awareness to be filled with the aroma of the beans being ground, and then the wafting of the brewing coffee smell. The task was to walk through all the elements of making and drinking coffee and to highlight ways he could use his senses to help him be present moment by moment. Like any meditation instructions, when he noticed his mind wandering to his to-do list for the day, ruminating thoughts about how exhausted and resentful he felt for having to get out of bed after another sleepless night, or some other thoughts that were about the past or future, he would notice that thinking had becoming the most dominant experience, and then he would allow the thoughts to drift into the background of his awareness and return to the present moment and whatever was actually happening in it. In this way, he was employing a skill that is extremely effective for addressing the universal issue of being in a constant state of distraction. He began to learn how to do what our dear friend and fellow mindfulness teacher (and creator of the mindfulness-based childbirth and parenting program) Nancy Bardacke says: "Start where you are, use what you have, do what you can, and minimize drama."

Years ago, another student who worked as a therapist stated: "I don't have time to sit (in meditation)." Yet in reality, she was actually "sitting" all the time. Whether it was a "meditation" or mindfulness practice or not depended on the quality of her attention, not the posture she was in or the actual activity she was doing. In fact, as a therapist, she was sitting for hours every day! By intentionally bringing a moment-to-moment nonjudgmental awareness to all the phenomena she was experiencing while she was with her clients (breath, sounds, sights, and so on), she could still develop mindful awareness. She could also take some time to be present for herself in between clients, even if for only ten or fifteen minutes at a time. (In fact, studies are mounting that indicate that even just a daily ten-minute practice of body and breath awareness can have significant effects on brain health, stress, and so on.)

The Buddha said meditation practice should be done sitting, standing, walking, and lying down. There is never a time when you not in one of those postures. So meditation or mindfulness can actually be practiced at any time.

Back in chapter 2, we introduced you to the "raisin meditation." This is a foundational practice offered in all official mindfulness-based interventions. While, in practice, it offers an experience of coming into closer contact with your senses, it is also an example of how to bring mindfulness into everyday activities. In our modern-day intensity-addicted society, where we're constantly on the lookout for something more exciting than the present moment to rescue us, the idea of deeply investigating the sensory nuances and direct experience of, say, tooth brushing or dish washing may seem somewhat absurd. But it is not.

As a mindfulness teacher, I (Catherine) am always exploring with people how they can weave moment-to-moment, nonjudgmental awareness seamlessly into their everyday lives. We can do "tooth brushing meditation," "dish washing meditation," "chopping vegetables meditation," "morning coffee drinking meditation," and on and on. In fact, anything you can think of that you already do, you can do mindfully, and make it a practice. Practices where we sit or lie down for a period of stillness while bringing a mindful attention to experiences such as the sensations of breath, other sensations in the body, sounds, the activity of thinking, and so on are what we call formal practices. An informal meditation is, well, everything else in our lives. The basic "instructions" for making something a "meditation" are exactly the same as if we were just sitting still: Become aware of the moment-to-moment sensory experiences, and when you notice the mind wandering into thoughts, stories, images about the past, the future, or anything else, simply notice this as "thinking," acknowledge that this is happening, and then bring your attention back to the direct sensory experiences of what is actually happening in the present moment.

Try it. See what activity of your daily life you can make into a "meditation."

But now it's time to practice the GMATI-1 meditation.

***

Now, return to your journal. Remembering that nonjudgment is at the heart of mindfulness, take a moment to reflect. What did you notice:

- In your body?

- In your mind?

- And in your mood?

Day 5: Learning to Pause

Today, we're going to continue on the theme of learning to develop present-moment awareness. To do this, you're going to learn a practical exercise that increases the "pause muscle." This ability to put yourself on "pause" is helpful because the more you are able to pause and increase the space between action and reaction, the more mindfulness you can cultivate and the more you will be able to move into the next moment with consciousness.

The point of meditation practice, both informal and formal, is not to just make you very good at sitting still. Or to make you stop thinking—as if *that* were possible. Nor is it actually about a quick fix to better sleep. It is, in fact, to become more conscious and aware of the expression of your own life as you're living it. To access the ability to be with your life with curiosity, friendliness, and intimacy. It is the only life you have, and this is the only moment you have to be in it. Peace comes with that. And with peace and a settling of mind and body comes deep rest.

As we've seen in previous chapters, the cultivation of mindfulness decreases the tension-filled reactivity that comes from being on autopilot. The less reactivity and more mindful engagement with life, the less likely the body is to be in a chronic state of flight/fight. So what we're really saying is that good sleep starts the moment you get out of bed. As you learn to settle down with yourself and the life that you have in this moment, your nervous system settles down, too.

This kind of seamlessness of mindfulness in everyday life also enables us to develop a deep friendship with ourselves. A friendship where there is understanding, accountability, compassion, and even humor. When we are paying attention, on purpose, in the present moment, and nonjudgmentally, we have the opportunity to uncover what our minds, emotions, and bodies are actually up to. We can begin to discover what is actually going on when we find ourselves in a state of irritability or avoidance. We may discover what thoughts were going through the mind that were triggering feelings of irritation, and what sensations of tightening or stress are in the body. Then we can pause, bring a compassionate and curious attention to ourselves, and just let it be. We can befriend ourselves by taking a deep breath, reminding ourselves of our humanity, and then perhaps making a conscious choice about how we want to respond to the next moment. This potent pause can benefit us in making decisions for how we communicate with others, what and how much we decide to put into our mouths, and so on.

> One practice, which I (Catherine) have been using for decades to teach people how to develop this ability to put ourselves on pause, is what I call the "yellow dot" exercise. It's called that because when I first started using it, I would give folks yellow dot stickers to place all around their

environment. They got placed on refrigerator doors, computer screens, bathroom mirrors, and so on. Whenever you see one of these visual reminders, the instructions are simply to:

1. Pause and take a breath, one that you are really present for.

2. And in that pause notice: "What is happening in the body right now?"

3. Also notice: "What thoughts are going through the mind? Am I in the future planning, or in the past rehashing?"

4. Also notice: "What emotions are present right now?"

5. Then, take another deep breath and go on your merry way.

   There is no need to change anything. You're simply strengthening the ability to pause and then nonjudgmentally notice.

Meditation Tip: Come Back Slowly

When you have finished your guided meditation, it's best to take a few moments to acknowledge your own effort to engage in meditation practice. It's not the best idea to just jump to your feet and start rushing around. Pause. Take a moment to stretch your body and visually take in your surroundings before returning to the activities of your daily life.

It's time again now to listen to and practice GMATI-1 meditation. Using the same idea of the pause while listening to the meditation, you can deepen your experience of being in contact with whatever is happening for you moment to moment.

***

Now take a moment to reflect and write in your journal. Remembering that nonjudgment is at the heart of mindfulness, what did you notice:

- In your body?

- In your mind?

- And in your mood?

Day 6: Deepening Attention on the Breath

It's been almost a week now that you have been practicing a meditation, where a lot of the time has been spent paying attention to the sensations of the breath. Today, we are going to take a deeper look into this seemingly mundane and yet extraordinary action that is keeping you alive. Using the breath as an anchor for the attention also helps to get some healthy distance from the power of the constantly thinking mind, with all of its enticing stories. Also, having more patience and acceptance with yourself and your own mind enables you to not take your own thinking and experiences so personally.

When we breathe in, we can experience an expanding and filling from the chest to the abdomen, and even into the back. If we're paying attention, we can also experience a kind of tickling in the nostrils as the air rushes past and enters the body. And as we breathe out, the reverse of the cycle happens. The breath is released as the chest cavity gets a bit smaller, causing the lungs to deflate as the breath moves back out through the nose.

It can be incredible to remember that this one breath, the one that is happening right now, contains oxygen that has been created in cooperation with the trees, as well as other gases that are part of our atmosphere. We draw in a breath and the body goes to work absorbing the oxygen into the bloodstream so that it can nourish all of the cells of our bodies. When we breathe out, carbon dioxide is offered back into the atmosphere, which is then picked up by the trees, because carbon dioxide is what they need in order to create oxygen. Each breath is a direct experience of our interconnectedness. Not just interconnectedness with the trees, but with all living breathing things. There is no such thing as *my* breath. But it is *the* breath that takes its turn uniting and intermingling with all life.

The breath is a friend, and is also a teacher. It is always teaching us how we can receive, and also how to let go. It is here, and then it is gone, just like everything else we can experience in a moment. By paying attention to the breath in this way, we also gain skill at paying attention to other body sensations, to sounds, and even to thoughts. Just like the breath, they are all impermanent. We can no more own a sound than we can own a breath or even a thought. They are not *mine,* but are simply the phenomena making up what we call this moment.

But the breath is also linked to how active the mind can be, as well as to the autonomic nervous system that regulates the fight and flight impulses as well as the relaxation response. When the breath is relaxed, even, and steady, the mind tends to follow. When we are stressed, the fight/flight system is active and the breath tends to be rapid and shallow. If we continue breathing rapidly, the body thinks it's still under threat and will keep the fight/flight system going. In contrast, notice what happens when you start to take some deep breaths. The stress response system begins to subside and turn itself down. The breath can act like a dial, either turning up the volume of the stress response when it is rapid and shallow, or turning it down when it is slow and steady.

Notice that you don't even always have to consciously slow down the breath. Simply bringing a kind and curious attention to its happening tends to slow it down and allow it to regulate itself all on its own. So today, as you listen to the meditation, bring your attention in close to what is actually happening as you breathe. Taste the breath, savor it, feel its rhythmic flow happening in and through you. Then see what happens when you move your attention to sounds, and then to thoughts. See if you can observe these other sensory experiences with the same kind and curious attention.

We've included a practice called the "three-minute breathing space." Feel free to use it during your day when things seem stressful and tense or whenever you want to do a brief mindfulness meditation. You might want to practice it now to see what it is like.

THREE-MINUTE BREATHING SPACE

This practice comes from the mindfulness-based cognitive therapy program (Segal, Williams, and Teasdale, 2002). It is very similar to what we introduced to you yesterday as the yellow dot exercise, except that it can be used any time and anywhere when things seem stressful and tense. It's called the "three-minute breathing space" because each of the three steps takes about a minute. It goes like this:

1. Start by putting yourself on pause and become aware of whatever thoughts, feelings, and sensations in the body are present. Let your awareness be broad, like a wide-angle lens, just observing what is showing up from one moment to the next.

2. Now, change the aperture of your awareness to focus in closely to the sensations of the breath. Particularly paying attention to the sensations of the breath in the nostrils, the chest, or the belly—letting thoughts, sounds, emotions, and body sensations (other than breath) all be in the background as you consistently redirect the focus of your attention back onto the direct experience of one breath at a time.

3. And now, broaden out the lens of your awareness again to feel your body as a whole—sitting or standing and feeling the whole body, the whole breath in the body.

    The image that's used in this practice is of an hourglass. You start with a broad view, like the wide opening at the top of the hourglass. That's the pause. Then you narrow the focus onto the breath, like the neck of the hourglass. This helps to anchor the mind, grounding it back into the present moment. Then, by opening the attention back up, like the bottom half of an hourglass, you open your awareness. Here, you are opening to life as it is, opening to yourself just as you are.

    This practice starts to train our attention to skillfully go from concentrated to expansive. The benefit is that in any automatic or multi-tasking moment, you begin to learn how to intentionally move your mind in order to step out of the demanding routines of autopilot. When we're caught up in our automatic reactions and routines, we're less likely to have nonjudgmental awareness. We're also less likely to be able to consciously and intentionally make choices about how we want to move into the next moment. It can also be of great help when we feel stressed or harried.

But now, once again, it's time to meditate using the GMATI-1 recording.

***

When you're finished, do some reflecting. Remembering that nonjudgment is at the heart of mindfulness, what did you notice:

- In your body?

- In your mind?

- And in your mood?

Day 7: Feeling Grounded

You are at the end of a whole week of mindfulness practice! Great job! Now, maybe you've noticed that sometimes, when you turn your attention to yourself, you can initially feel somewhat emotionally overwhelmed. This is not uncommon. It's not that easy to stop in the middle of a busy life and turn toward your own mind and heart. If this is happening for you, the following is a practice that we find extremely helpful for settling and grounding. When we're exhausted and anxiety arises, we may feel unsettled and even unsafe. When we are caught in the grips of thinking about all that we believe will go wrong in the future, or what is wrong with us now, we need a safe harbor and anchor to rest in. So try this exercise:

If you are sitting down, make sure you place both feet on the floor. Then:

1. Rub your feet back and forth on the floor to activate that sense of connection with the ground.

2. Now, come to a standing position and feel the soles of the feet on the floor.

3. Begin to notice the sensations of contact that your feet are making with the floor.

4. To better feel these sensations, try gently rocking forward and backward on your feet, and then side to side. Perhaps making little circles with your knees so that you feel how sensations in the feet change depending on where you place your weight.

5. Whenever you notice the mind has wandered into thoughts, just return the attention again to the sensations at the soles of your feet.

6. Now, take a step forward and notice the sensations changing in the soles of the feet. Become aware of the foot lifting off the floor, stepping forward, and then taking the whole of

your weight as you shift onto it. Then doing the same thing with the other foot.

7. Take a few steps, one foot after the other, and notice what you feel.

8. As you walk, you can even bring in a sense of appreciation for how small the surface areas of the feet are, and how your feet support your entire body. If you wish, you can even allow a moment of gratitude for the hard work your feet do for you every day, which we often take for granted.

9. Just continue taking a few steps, noticing the soles of the feet.

10. Now, return to standing still once again. Expand your awareness to your entire body, letting yourself feel whatever you're feeling and letting yourself be just as you are.

Meditation Tip: A Little Ceremony Can Help

Some people find that they can enhance their guided meditation by establishing a little "ceremony."

Start with a few minutes to compose yourself and invite your body into a state of ease. Turn off your cell phone, close any doors, and place pets outside the area where you are meditating. You might even develop a ritual in which you light a candle or ring a bell to signify the start of your practice, and then ring the bell again and extinguish the candle at the end, to mark the transition to other activities in your life.

Of course, these particular steps aren't essential. Guided meditations are not dependent on ceremony. But when you carve out and distinguish your mindset for formal practice, you boost your intention for practice and delineate the time as special.

You don't even have to use just the feet to do this kind of "grounding" practice. If you're sitting while reading this, take a moment to feel your bottom making contact with whatever you are resting on. Tune in to the sensations of contact—the pressure, warmth, softness, or hardness. Feel how much of your body is touching the surface of the chair or couch. You can then put your feet on the floor if they're not there already and feel your contact with the earth. These solid surfaces are holding you.

Feeling safe and grounded and in our bodies helps us in so many ways. We often use the expression "I'm going out of my mind" to describes states of anxiety or stress. It's a great statement because it points to something important. Although we aren't really "out of our minds," we *are* out of our mindfulness. We're being flooded with thoughts and emotions and are getting totally disconnected from our bodies. We need a way to get back.

When we're out of our mindfulness, we don't think straight or make clear decisions. (This is even more likely to happen if we have a sleep-deprived, muddled mind.) What happens then is that we mostly react. We tend to get impulsive and just grab for whatever will bring immediate relief.

So as you work to carve out the time to do the GMATI meditations and other formal mindfulness practices in this book, also remember: Mindful presence is available right now. All you need to do is *be.*

***

Start today's practice of GMATI-1 meditation by really paying attention to all that supports you and helps you feel grounded. Then, when you have finished the meditation, do some reflecting.

Remembering that nonjudgment is at the heart of mindfulness, what did you notice:

- In your body?
- In your mind?
- And in your mood?

Congratulations! You have completed the first week of GMATI. You are now ready to move on to the rest of the GMATI sequence that will greatly improve your sleep.

CHAPTER 5

GMATI—Week 2

Welcome to GMATI Week 2! After simply becoming *aware* of your sleep and the emotions that accompany it in Week 1, the emphasis this week will be on *accepting or allowing* your sleep to be exactly as it is, rather than directly trying to change it. Acceptance is dependent on first being aware, then seeing if you can just allow whatever is happening to be there without trying to evaluate it or change it. This is a really crucial skill in mindfulness practice, but it is something that we need to practice, because it doesn't come naturally. It's natural to want to change what we don't like. But sometimes, we can't change it, and then the most compassionate thing we can do for ourselves is learn to accept it.

By learning the GMATI-2 practice, which is primarily a body scan meditation, you'll increase your ability to practice acceptance of sensations, emotions, and reactions in general and apply that ability to your insomnia. And in so doing, you'll be changing your *relationship* to your sensations, emotions, and reactions. You'll also get to learn some other ways to bring relaxation into your body; some additional formal mindfulness practices; some self-compassion practices;

how to use imagery to support your meditation; and affectionate breathing.

Note: It is best not to proceed with this chapter until you have had at least a full week of practice with the GMATI-1 guided meditation and are comfortable with it. If not, then continue practicing GMATI-1 until you are ready to move on to Week 2.

Here's an initial way to start learning how to exercise your "allowing" muscle: Read through this week's meditation first before practicing so that you become familiar with the instructions and begin to mentally "download" the kind of guidance that supports the experience of "allowing." But remember, reading is not the same thing as practicing! You need to actually listen to the recording and practice it daily to fully "exercise" this learning.

Just like with GMATI-1, you need to find a comfortable place for your practice. You can use the sitting postures we showed you in Week 1, or even better, you can lie down to do this practice. In the GMATI-2 meditation, which takes about twenty-five minutes to practice, you will be learning to pay attention to sensations in the body, and by lying down, you can be in an open posture where often more sensations are noticeable. However, it's *very* important that, for now, you not do this practice in your bed. If you choose to practice it lying down, put some cushioning on the floor to support your head and other bony parts of the body that may need some softness to support them. You may also want to place a cushion under your knees to support your lower back.

Important Tip

For the time being, *do not* practice mindfulness meditation at night to try to fall asleep or as a relaxation strategy. Rather, do guided meditation during your normal waking hours. You then don't have to do anything more. Let the guided meditation work for you by changing how you perceive your sleep, and thereby indirectly improve it. It is that simple.

Here is this week's meditation for you to read now:

GMATI-2

Begin by getting into a position lying on your back or sitting in a chair. Allow the legs and arms to be loose alongside your body. Let the weight of your body be supported by the gravity that brings you in contact with the surface you are resting on. Become aware of the places in which your body makes contact with the floor, bed, or chair, and allow yourself to settle in fully.

Start by taking a few moments to welcome yourself into this time and place—a time you have carved out for yourself to let go of the mode that we all find ourselves in. Switch from a mode of doing, evaluating, planning for the future, and rehashing the past, and into a mode of simple being. Of just being in the present moment as it is, knowing there is no place to go right now, nothing to do. Release all effort for doing, all trying. Allow yourself to just be aware of being right here and right now. Open to the experience of sensing directly what is present, with no need to try to analyze or problem solve. It may be helpful to think of this as a time for you. A time for simply being with yourself and letting be.

And now notice that without your having to do anything in particular, you are breathing. Notice the sensations of the breath as it enters the body, and as it leaves the body. Notice the breath making subtle movements in your abdomen as you breathe in and out, as the belly expands on the inhalation and then softens on the exhalation.

Breathe in and know that you are breathing in. Breathe out and know you are breathing out. You may even want to place your hands on the abdomen to feel the gentle rise and fall of the breath as it moves in and out. Simply allow the breath to enter and leave the body of its own accord, without changing it or trying to control it in any way. Ride the waves of your breathing in the belly. You don't have to do anything or to be in any particular way. Simply allow the breath to breathe itself.

Notice each inhale and each exhale. Focus the awareness of the breath and the abdomen. Feel the belly expanding on the inhalation, contracting on the exhalation. Be mindful of breathing in and breathing out. No need to control; simply breathing normally and breathing naturally, moment to moment. Breathing in and breathing out. Being aware. Controlling only our awareness. Breathing is all there is.

Also, feel how you are holding yourself in the body. Just accept this, feeling any physical sensations—sensations of warmth, coolness, tightness, softening, itching, gripping, and just letting them be. Just acknowledging what is being felt; just allowing it.

When you notice that the mind has wandered into thoughts, memories, stories about what is happening, gently congratulate yourself for being aware of this experience. You may also notice thoughts about the thoughts. Just gently and compassionately acknowledge wherever the mind has wandered, perhaps making a mental note: "wandering," and just making room for the thoughts as they come and go. Then, gently escort yourself back to a sense of the body breathing—the breath in and the breath out.

You may notice the mind labeling thoughts and emotions with evaluations such as "bad" or "getting worse." If so, try thanking the mind for the label and return to the present experience as it is, without needing it to be other than what it is. You can even call those thoughts "thinking" and neutralize the perception of "good and bad."

As best you can, also bring the attitude of generous allowance and gentle acceptance to the rest of your experience. There is nothing to be fixed, no particular state to be achieved. Simply allow the experience to be your experience, with no need to be other than what it is.

As we move into a body scan, if at any time certain sensations in the body become too strong or uncomfortable, or if emotions arise that feel too difficult, know that you can always return to the sensations of the breath. Return to the breath as an anchor, as a way of stabilizing your attention; doing this until you are ready to resume the body scan.

Now, move your attention all the way down to your toes and notice: What can be felt here?

Now, as you progressively move your attention through your body, explore being present for each of the regions listed below and any sensations you may find in them. As you do this, you are practicing simple awareness. You are acknowledging what is already there and letting it be. Try to just notice the sensations with curiosity and kindness, and when you notice that your mind has taken you elsewhere, remind yourself to keep coming back to the ongoing flow of sensations that are alive in the body.

- Start by moving your attention all the way down to your toes and notice: What can be felt here? Now slowly, one at a time, bring this awareness into your:

Feet

Ankles

Calves and shins

Knees

Thighs

Hips

Buttocks/pelvis

Lower back

Middle of the back

Upper back and shoulders

Abdomen

Chest

Heart

Return to the shoulders

Upper arms

Lower arms

Hands and fingers

Neck—both front and back

Jaw

Cheeks

Nose

Eyes

Ears

The sides of the head

The back of the head

The top of the head

This journey through the body is about feeling into the body, becoming acquainted with the sensations of aliveness, comfort, discomfort, about being mindful of any sensations that arise. Acknowledging their presence and then letting whatever arises go, wherever it needs to go. Just being present. Noticing the changing nature of bodily sensations—how they come and go. Don't try to hold on to any body sensations or to make them go away. Just accept them and let them be.

Now, gently expanding your awareness to the body as a whole, just be present here in the body, breathing.... And now, turn your attention to any emotions or thoughts that may be present right now, noticing that like body sensations, even thoughts and emotions can come and go, they too are ever changing. Just be present with the thinking and the feeling, realizing that *you* are not necessarily your thoughts or emotions, no matter how insistent or persistent they may be. Just include them as a part of your practice of simply being aware of what is arising, acknowledging their presence and then letting them be or letting them go as they will.

And now, we'll use these last few moments as an opportunity to explore any thoughts or emotions specifically around your sleep. Bring to mind any thoughts about your sleep and see what emotions arise. Be present with what may be within you as you feel into these thoughts and accept them just as they are, without the need to change them or make them go away. You might be experiencing some frustration, fears, or worries about your sleep. The invitation here is to put your attention into your direct experience of being worried or sad or frustrated about your sleep. You can do this by first noticing and even labeling the emotion—*"Frustration is here"*—and then allowing yourself to feel any accompanying sensations in the body.

Maybe there is a tightening in the jaw, throat, chest, or belly. Maybe there is a welling up, or pressure in the chest as frustration turns into sadness. Or maybe there is nothing at all. Just allow yourself to feel and acknowledge whatever it is that you are feeling. Know that there is nothing that you need to do, such as analyzing or trying to figure out why you feel this way. Rather, just feel the feeling of the worry, the frustration, the sadness of not sleeping the way you would like, accept it, and just let it be. Feeling whatever there is to be felt, noticing what arises in the mind when you think about your sleep. Noticing any reactions in the body and just acknowledging whatever comes up, then letting it be.

Now, gently withdraw from the practice of mindfully inquiring about thoughts and feelings relating to sleep, and come back to feeling the body as a whole. Notice the abdomen rising up on inhalation and falling on exhalation. Feel yourself connected from head to toe and to fingertips; feel the body as a whole. Breathing in and breathing out.

As you breathe in and out, just let whatever is being felt ripple and resonate; let it be. Acknowledge things as they are.

Now, take these last few moments to feel some gratitude toward yourself for having made this effort for your health and well-being. You've taken time to simply be present with your experience as it is without the need to make it any different, without the need to do anything except to be aware and to simply be present.

Now, begin to gently bring your attention back to the place where you are, and to the activities of your day. Recognize that this feeling of presence, of focus, that you have just experienced is as close as the next moment—as close as the next breath.

Day 1: The Nature of Sensations

Welcome to the first day of Week 2. As you practice the body scan, you are developing the capacity to pay attention to sensations in the body through a mindful perspective—meaning just observing without judgment. As you do this, you may start to notice a few themes:

Sensations Are Not Static

They are impermanent and always changing. An itch, for example, may start off in a concentrated way with some intensity. Eventually, it passes and ceases to be.

Sensations Are Multifaceted

One sensation may actually consist of a number of different feelings. Take that itch again. It may consist of tingling, scratching, stabbing, prickling. It can rise in intensity and then can spread and change as it progresses.

Sensations Capture the Attention

Physical sensations give the mind something more concrete to pay attention to. However, we are used to turning away from sensations in the body, especially if they are unpleasant. So we need to discover all the ways in which we lose touch with our own bodies, and how, through mindfulness, we can return. We return, with kindness, to just noticing moment to moment what is actually here.

There are many reasons that learning how to be more tuned in to the body can be healing. One is that if we are disconnected from our bodies, we lessen our ability to make wise and kind choices about how to take care of the body. Another is that by becoming more aware of the arising sensations in the body, we can actually become more skillful at being in touch with and working with our emotions. It's actually true that whenever we have an emotion—joy, sadness, frustration, anger, delight—different feelings arise in the body that go along with the emotion. By becoming more familiar with the sensations in the body that accompany an emotion, we get better at being able to stay with our emotions, rather than reacting to them or even believing them to be permanent, or that they are a problem, or that they define who we are. But remember that we need a lot of patience and kindness to do this practice.

For example, when you recognize that you are feeling "frustrated" because you are not able to sleep, pause for a moment and see what "frustration" actually feels like. Do you notice any tightening in muscles, heat, cold, constriction, heaviness, or pressure?

If so, instead of doing the usual thing of dwelling on what your mind is saying about *why* you feel frustrated or zooming into the future and assuming you'll be frustrated for a long time, just *pause.* Just notice what the sensations actually are, in exactly the same way that you're learning to do with the body scan.

When you experience the physical sensations of "frustration" because of your thoughts and feelings about the frustration, you can "uncouple" them from thoughts and emotions by bringing a kind and curious awareness to the sensations themselves. You could even imagine breathing into the sensation as a way of offering yourself some comfort and support for staying with the sensation. And see what happens. You could even gently and silently say to yourself: "Oh, frustration *feels* like this." By naming the experience, you make it much easier to actually deal with. There is a saying that you "name it to tame it."

You can also try expanding your attention around the sensations into areas of the body where there is little or no sensation, or to a place where the feelings are neutral, and know that this too is happening in the present moment and that there is really more to you than just the *frustration* that is present. When you do this, you are embodying the very important and healing attitude of *allowing.*

It's time now to practice with the GMATI-2 meditation.

***

When you are through, you might want to pause and ask yourself: "What did I discover when doing this meditation?" Go ahead and jot down in your journal some things that you noticed happening for you. Now, remembering that nonjudgment is at the heart of mindfulness, what did you notice:

- In your body?

- In your mind?

- And in your mood?

Day 2: Allowing

The earlier chapters of this book described chronic insomnia as a "vicious cycle," when poor sleep leads to emotional arousal or agitation, which in turn causes more poor sleep, which in turn causes more emotional arousal and agitation, and so on. That's exhausting just to write! This whole process takes a lot of energy, which makes you feel even more tired than if you were simply awake without struggle. As you may be beginning to find out, trying to control your sleep can end up making things even worse.

Mindful awareness can help break this vicious cycle. In Week 1, we had you start by simply being *aware* of your struggle with sleep and the emotions that accompany it, but not evaluating these things. This week, we are emphasizing the next aspect of mindfulness—that of *allowing* or *accepting* what your sleep is like, and the emotions that accompany it.

Allowing enables you to stop being "at war" with yourself and your experiences. Mindfulness practice invites you to be an observer who simply notices your sleep and accompanying body sensations, thoughts, and emotions as *things*—things that are not who you are, but just something you are experiencing—and to just accept them as they are.

This might seem like you are giving up and giving in to your insomnia; that you are "resigning" yourself to a life of insomnia. But in fact, this is not passive resignation, but active acceptance. Resignation is a negative state that involves being stuck where you are and not doing anything. Acceptance is a positive act whereby you are purposefully choosing to just acknowledge what you observe. It is recognition that if something already is the way it is, it only creates suffering to struggle with it. If it's already part of the present moment, it doesn't do us any good to deny that it exists. When we accept what is here, we are subscribing or consenting to reality.

This in no way implies that it will always be that way. Accepting that you have a problem with insomnia is the most essential step to sleeping naturally. It changes your attitude to and your relationship with sleep. Your sleep is not bad; it just is what it is. It may not be comfortable or feel good to you, and it is most certainly not your preference. But accepting it or allowing it as it is showing up in this moment reduces the need to struggle to change your sleep. It also reduces the stress and anxiety that can accompany your poor sleep. You simply observe your lack of sleep and the emotions that accompany it without evaluation and without trying to change anything. As you will see, in the end, this will actually begin to improve the quality and then the quantity of your sleep.

What's in a Word

Language, and the way we talk to ourselves and others, is really crucial here. In the English language, we use the verb "to be" to describe states that are in reality transient. We say "I *am* tired," "I *am* frustrated," or "I *am* an insomniac," but it would be more accurate to say "I'm feeling or experiencing fatigue/frustration/insomnia, etc." Other languages do a better job at this. In other languages, one might say "I have..." to reveal feelings or states of being. This is much more accurate, much more in line with the way things actually are.

This is related to how we think about things, too, and the relationship we have to our own thoughts. There is a difference between being *in* a thought and *observing* a thought. If you think, "I'm an insomniac," you are *in* that thought and are likely to feel bad. It can seem like that is all you are; it is your total being. But if you notice that you are thinking, "I have insomnia," then you are just observing that thought without being caught up in it or overly identified with it. Furthermore, it is just one thought among many;

just a part of a whole host of thoughts that might make up the kaleidoscope of the mind. But it is *not* who you are.

Think back before you had a problem with insomnia. You probably never even thought much about sleep. But now, you can't seem to stop thinking about it. This is perfectly natural, but not necessary, and surely not helpful. As we showed in chapter 3, sleep is a regulated natural physiological process that requires no conscious effort or energy for it to occur, just like the beating of your heart.

In order for you to learn how to simply notice, and to accept your sleep the way it is and not try to change it, you will need:

- A willingness to give up your efforts to control your sleep.

- A willingness to simply allow the experiencing of thoughts, feelings, and bodily sensations that accompany your sleep problem.

- And a huge boatload of compassion for yourself, for being a human being who is suffering in this way.

Likewise, you need to accept that there are things about your insomnia that you cannot change, such as your possible genetic propensity for somewhat less than optimal sleep, past events that triggered your insomnia, and the thoughts and emotions that accompany your poor sleep. What you can control is how you *relate* to your insomnia and all that accompanies it.

Mindfulness encourages you to be willing to be aware of your sleep as it is, and then accept it as it is. Acceptance is an act of compassion and of nonviolence with yourself. Acceptance means that you choose not to struggle with your poor sleep and all the pain and suffering that comes with it. Rather, you accept that at times you cannot sleep as well as you would like to. You accept that unwanted thoughts come to mind when you attempt to sleep. You accept the stress and anxiety that poor sleep causes. That is, what you change is not the sleep itself but your *relationship* to sleep and its consequences. After you begin to change this relationship, you will notice an improvement in the quality of your sleep, and later, you will also see an increase in the quantity of sleep you get.

Learning to mindfully acknowledge and allow whatever is happening with your sleep requires fierce compassion, as well as putting in the time to meditate with discipline and consistency. The more you practice mindfulness, the greater will be your decrease in agitation and arousal, which in turn will help you sleep better.

Okay, with all the kindness you can muster, it's time to practice the GMATI-2 meditation again.

***

When you are finished, take a few minutes to reflect. Now, remembering that nonjudgment is at the heart of mindfulness, what did you notice:

- In your body?

- In your mind?

- And in your mood?

Day 3: Stretching into Relaxation

Today we will be doing a little stretching or mindful movement before practicing with the GMATI-2 meditation. In this practice, you will be nourishing, strengthening, and relaxing your body, and participating in the process of optimizing your state of well-being and health. Pay close attention to the experience of *release* after doing a stretch. This simple awareness can teach you a lot about what it feels like to "relax" your body. (You may also start to see the relationship of relaxation in the body to relaxation in the mind—that is, to the practice of *allowing* in the mind.)

You will find a guided recording for this stretching practice on the New Harbinger website: http://www.newharbinger.com/42587. We encourage you to read the instructions through first, imagining your body doing each of the stretches, so that when you do practice, you know what's coming. Just follow along as best you can, doing what is possible for you and refraining from anything that does not seem to be appropriate or that is painful for you at this time.

MINDFUL STRETCHING PRACTICE

In the process of developing a deeper awareness and sensitivity to yourself, you may be working at the limits of what you can do at any given moment. It's important to be aware of these limits, and to dwell at their boundary long enough to experience them, but not to go beyond them. Let your own sensitivity to your body override these instructions as to how *long* to hold any position you may be doing. Rather, look deeply into each moment with full acceptance, not forcing yourself to be different than you are right now.

Additionally, when doing these stretches, if you wish or need to stop doing a particular stretch or are unable to do it, try instead assuming a comfortable posture, closing your eyes, and visualizing yourself sensing or doing what the recording is describing in as much detail as possible. Remember to allow yourself to breathe fully and freely. Work with your eyes open sometimes, with your eyes closed sometimes. Allow yourself to experiment and explore, noticing your changing levels of concentration.

1.   Start by either sitting in a chair or standing up. Take a moment to feel the sensations of contact

you are making with whatever solid surfaces are supporting you.

2. With an uplifted spine, allow your head to bend forward, bringing your chin down toward your chest. Feel any sensations of stretching at the back of your neck, or even down your back. Take a few breaths here and continue to feel the sensations in this posture.

3. Lift your head back up and pause for a moment. What sensations are present now?

4. Let your right ear tilt down toward your right shoulder and allow the heaviness of your head to create feelings of stretching on the left side of your neck. Breathe here for a few moments to just feel what there is to feel. Then lift your head back up, and repeat on the other side.

5. When you bring your head back up again, pause to see what you notice in your neck and shoulders.

6. At this point, try slowly and gently swinging your head from side to side with the head bent forward in the middle, opening up and stretching the back of the neck. When you're through, go back to your starting position and let your head rest on the top of your neck.

7. Now, draw both shoulders up toward your ears in a big shrug, and then squeeze your shoulder blades together and draw the shoulders back.

Then, drop them down before bringing them forward to complete one shoulder roll. Do this a few times in each direction. When you are through, just pause and notice what sensations are present in your neck and shoulders.

8. Now, let both of your arms start to float out from your sides, slowly and mindfully raising the arms up above your head and reaching toward the ceiling. Stretch one side upward and then the other, as if you were picking apples off of a tree. Notice the sensations of stretching through the arms, the shoulders, down each side of your body, and even down into the back.

9. After going from side to side a few times, *very* slowly start to let the arms float back down toward your sides. Take your time, and feel the changing nature of sensations as the arms recruit different muscles to support and stabilize this movement. Feel when the arms get very heavy, and then finally, when they reach the point where they are back down along your sides, feel the release of the work you just did.

10. Pause, and breathe with this feeling of release.

11. Now, let your head come back down toward your chest, and then start to let the whole upper body round forward, bringing your upper torso toward your thighs. If you are standing, make sure to bend your knees so that the upper body can just hang forward like a rag doll.

12. After a few moments of hanging forward and breathing, slowly start to unfurl the spine, bringing it back upward. Pause and feel the sensations that are present with this movement.

13. Now, take a few deep breaths. Maybe taking a moment to appreciate your body and whatever ability it has right now to engage in these gentle stretches. Knowing that whatever you experienced is what you experienced. There is no perfect place to get to. Appreciating even your intention to stretch and bring this kind of caring in to your body.

Is a stretch producing sensations of pulling or tugging or warmth or tingling or something else? Try to notice precisely what you are feeling, even ask yourself: "What am I feeling now? What is this feeling in my neck, my shoulders, or my arms? *Exactly* where is it? What qualities does this feeling have? Is my mind reacting or responding to the feelings?"

If you continue to do this with *care,* attention, and regularity, you will soon notice that your limits are changing, and dissolving, by themselves. The best effort is effort involving patience, acceptance, and consistency. The finest results will be achieved by not trying to achieve anything at all, even relaxation. It's enough to simply do what the stretching recording says to do, as best you can, paying full attention to how *your* body is feeling in *each* moment.

Now it's time to practice the GMATI-2 meditation.

***

Afterward, take a few minutes to reflect and jot down some things in your journal that you noticed in your meditation today. Now, remembering that nonjudgment is at the heart of mindfulness, what did you notice:

- In your body?

- In your mind?

- And in your mood?

Day 4: Easing into a Full Breath

Today, as you begin to read in preparation for practicing, let's have you try doing something that will help bring some ease into your body. Notice the area around your eyes and your forehead and allow the muscles there to soften—like butter melting in the sun. Now, do the same thing at your jaw ... and your neck ... and your shoulders, just letting all tension drain out of those areas. Now, start to feel the space around your heart melting and softening, and then bring that same sense of ease into your belly, hips, and pelvis—letting all these areas melt a little and release any extra holding that isn't necessary for sitting where you are in this moment.

When you start a meditation by intentionally bringing some ease into your body, you are helping to set the stage for allowing and acceptance. You can also do this by purposefully deepening your breath with diaphragmatic breathing as you start to practice.

DIAPHRAGMATIC BREATHING

Think of your chest as a flexible five-gallon rubber bottle with a hole at the top. Inside this rubber bottle are two balloons. Each balloon is connected to a tube. The two tubes merge into a single tube that goes through the otherwise airtight narrow opening at the top of the bottle. The balloons inflate when walls of the rubber bottle are stretched, causing the volume of the rubber bottle to increase, creating a partial vacuum. The opposite happens when the volume of the bottle decreases. These processes alternate over and over again, causing air to flow into the balloons and then to be forced out. This is how we breathe in and then breathe out.

We inhale when the chest expands to increase its volume. The chest can expand in two different ways. One way is by little muscles between the individual ribs changing the positioning of the ribs such that the chest expands. The second way is when the diaphragm (the domelike muscle that is the floor of the chest) flattens, which also tends to push the belly out as well as increase the volume of the chest. We exhale when the opposite occurs.

Typically, when we are standing or sitting upright we breathe by expanding and contracting our rib cage.

But we can instead, if we choose to, breathe by flattening the diaphragm. This type of breathing is inherently more relaxing.

It can be helpful to know how to do diaphragmatic breathing at the beginning of a meditation. Start by placing one hand on your upper chest and the other on your abdomen. When you are upright and breathing normally you will probably notice the chest expanding, but not much change at the belly. This time, allow your stomach to swell forward as if the air is filling it. As you breathe out, allow the stomach to gently fall back, as if the air is now leaving it. Meanwhile, there's probably little or no movement in your chest. Without exaggerating any of these movements, try slowing your breathing down a bit and take slightly bigger or deeper breaths when doing diaphragmatic breathing. You may also want to rest briefly in the pause at the end of the exhale before breathing in again. Eventually, you can just adopt a pace and depth of breathing that feels comfortable for you.

AFFECTIONATE BREATHING

Now that you have been able to experience practicing deeper and fuller breaths, let the breath return to its natural rhythm. Then perk up the attention on it and how it feels in the body by warming up your awareness with affectionate breathing.

1. As you continue to feel your breath in your body, try internally inclining toward it as if you were greeting a beloved friend or a dear child.

2. Try very slightly turning up the corners of your mouth, as if you had just the very beginnings of a smile coming across your face.

3. Feel how each breath nourishes you, and allow yourself to be internally caressed by the breath. As each breath comes in and your body expands, and then as it leaves on the exhale and you feel the release of the expansion in your chest and belly, feel the gentle rocking sensations that the breath creates within you.

4. You are being nourished, rocked, and caressed by each breath. And so, greet each breath with tenderness and affection.

   This practice is adapted from the *Mindful Self-Compassion Workbook* by Kristin Neff and Christopher Germer (2018).

Now it's time to practice the GMATI-2 meditation again. Try bringing in some diaphragmatic breathing and warming up your attention with an attitude of affection.

***

When you are finished, take a few minutes to return to your journal. Remembering that nonjudgment is at the heart of mindfulness, what did you notice:

- In your body?

- In your mind?

- And in your mood?

Day 5: Introduction to Self-Compassion

At this point in the practice, you may be finding you need additional support in learning to befriend yourself as you learn to accept your sleep and yourself just as you are. Because, let's face it, you may be finding that being a good friend to yourself while you are struggling is not easy. While presence and allowing are innate capacities, they are not always easy to access and they may not feel natural. Human beings have a lot of training and experience in living with a constantly distracted mind, as well as in resisting things that are unpleasant. Life is full of difficult experiences that help to forge a shell of armor around our hearts. The human heart is both incredibly resilient and profoundly tender and vulnerable. When we are not feeling at ease and safe, we contract and resist. In mindfulness practice, you are exercising a different mode—one that is about opening and allowing. You may feel frustrated with it and a little wobbly in trying to practice in it.

In day 2 of this week, we looked at mindfulness and how mindful awareness enables us to "see" and encounter things the way they are. Many teachings on mindful awareness describe it as a bird. The two wings of awareness are *clear seeing* and *compassion.* Both are required to make the bird of mindful awareness fly. If we just focus on the bare engagement with life through clear seeing we can become embittered. It's too raw. We need compassion to enable us to be with things as they are. So today, we will introduce you to mindful self-compassion and provide instructions for practices that can be used by themselves and in combination with the GMATI meditations.

The Dalai Lama defines the word compassion as "the trembling of the heart in the face of suffering along with the desire to help soothe and alleviate the suffering." As mammals, we are hardwired for this kind of response to others. This hardwiring is why we rally around our friends and even strangers in times of hardship and difficulty. It's also why we feel resonance even with characters in a movie, and why witnessing their suffering makes us cry.

But what about when we're the ones experiencing the difficulty? Like, say, the difficulty of not being able to sleep, and the physical depletion and mental fogginess we feel as a result of insomnia. Where is compassion then?

PRACTICE: HOW DO YOU TREAT A FRIEND?

To understand this a little more, try this practice the *Mindful Self-Compassion Workbook* adapted from Kristin Neff and Christopher Germer (2018).

Take out a piece of paper, but first reflect before you write.

Think for a moment about a friend you may know now, or knew in the past, who struggled in some way. Maybe she failed a test, maybe she was going through a breakup, maybe she lost her job, maybe her health was compromised, or maybe she, too, struggled with insomnia. She was hurting, felt inadequate, and was suffering in some way. Take out a piece of paper and jot down the answers to these questions:

How did you treat her?

What words of comfort did you use?

How did you address her?

What was your tone of voice?

What kind of body language did you use?

Now, reflect again. Think about a time when *you* were struggling. You failed at something, lost something, made a mistake, or felt inadequate and were suffering in some way. Take out another piece of paper and jot down the answers to these questions:

How did you treat yourself?

What words of comfort did you use?

How did you address yourself?

What was your tone of voice?

What kind of body language did you use?

Did you notice any difference? If you did, you are not alone. Neff found that (in the US at least) the vast majority of people are significantly more compassionate toward others than themselves (Neff and Germer, 2018). Only a very few people are more compassionate to themselves than others, and the rest are about equal in their compassion.

In chapter 1, we looked at how the threat-defense system works in our bodies (our reptilian brain). It's a system that, when triggered, releases cortisol and adrenaline to get us ready to fight, flee, or freeze. But when we feel depleted, broken, or inadequate, the "threat" is about our sense of self and we sometimes attack the problem—ourselves!

Luckily, along with our reptile remnants, we are also mammals. And because mammalian young are born immature and need an extended time of nurturance, we are also hardwired for a kind of caregiving that keeps infants safe and close to their care-givers. This mammalian care-giving system is triggered by two main factors—soothing touch and gentle vocalizations (Steller and Keltner, 2014). These factors release oxytocin and opiates in both parents and children, helping the infant feel safe and secure.

Think about the various ingredients that are necessary when feeling compassion toward others. When those we care about are suffering, we first notice it. Then we respond with kindness and we attempt to help them feel connected. We may reach out and hug them, put a hand on a shoulder, or do something similar. In doing this, we are bringing warmth and soothing. We tend to change the tone of our voice or even make nonverbal vocalizations to signify our care. We may also say words of soothing comfort to let them know we are there to support them. These are the same ingredients needed for self-compassion.

Self-compassion is simply treating ourselves with the same kindness, warmth, and care that we would treat a friend when things go wrong. When you give youself compassion, especially accompanied by physical gestures of self-compassion such as placing a hand over your heart, on your belly, or any other place that feels soothing, you are activating that same mammalian safety response, and in so doing, you are counteracting the stress generated by the threat-defense system.

Keeping in mind this possibility of befriending yourself with compassion, it's now time to practice the GMATI-2 meditation again.

***

As before, when you are finished, take a few minutes to write in your journal. Now, remembering that nonjudgment is at the heart of mindfulness, what did you notice:

- In your body?

- In your mind?

- And in your mood?

Day 6: Practicing Self-Compassion

Yesterday, we spent a little time exploring the differences between how we treat a friend and how we treat ourselves. Today, you are going to deepen your understanding of self-compassion and experience a practice that will enable you to directly apply compassion to yourself when you are struggling.

Self-Compassion Model

Kristin Neff (2003) created a template for self-compassion that has these three components:

- Mindfulness

- Common humanity

- Self-kindness

In order for us to bring compassion to ourselves when we are suffering, we first need to know that we are suffering. *Mindfulness* enables us to nonjudgmentally turn toward ourselves and really get a sense of what is happening in the present moment. It enables us to see things clearly without swinging to the extremes of either avoiding what we are feeling or getting carried away into a dramatic storyline of our current situation.

Once we see what's here, we can open our perspective and remember that *all human beings struggle and experience difficulty.* This is our common humanity. It's what we share, not what makes us different. No one is perfect. So when we struggle or fail at something, it's common to feel as though we are the only one in the world who is suffering in this way. You may know rationally that this is not true, but when you're in the middle of insomnia, for example, it's easy to imagine that everyone else is sleeping soundly—and to feel isolated and disconnected from your fellow humans. This "emotional tunnel vision" isn't a logical process, says psychologist Kristin Neff. "You become absorbed by your own feelings of insufficiency and insecurity. When you're in the confined space of self-loathing, it's as if the rest of humanity doesn't even exist."

The result, frequently, is intense feelings of loneliness and despair. Thoughts like, *Why is this happening to me?* further intensify the pain of the experience. "The emotion of compassion springs from the recognition that the human experience is imperfect, that we are all fallible," says Dr. Neff. "Why else would we say, 'It's only human' to comfort someone who has made a mistake? When we're in touch with our common humanity, we remember that feelings of inadequacy and disappointment are universal. This is what distinguishes self-compassion from self-pity. While self-pity says 'poor me,' self-compassion recognizes suffering is part of the shared human experience. The pain I feel in difficult times is the same pain that you feel in difficult times. The triggers are different, the circumstances are different, the degree of pain is different, but the basic experience is the same" (2018).

It's called being human! Join the club.

When it comes to insomnia, it's important to keep in mind that you're not alone. As Dr. Neff notes, many circumstances of our lives, and even aspects of ourselves, are not of our intentional choosing, "but instead stem from innumerable factors that are outside our sphere of influence. When we acknowledge this reality, failings and life difficulties do not have to be taken so personally" (2018).

And lastly, we learn to *treat ourselves with kindness,* care, understanding, discernment, and support—just like we would treat someone we care about. We actively soothe ourselves with internal messages (after all, we're talking to ourselves all the time anyway!). We utilize a friendly and warm tone to address ourselves, and the result is the creation of a good friendship with ourselves. Some even refer to self-compassion as being your own "inner ally."

When the threat-defense system gets turned inward, fight manifests as self-criticism, flight as self-isolation, and freeze as self-absorption or rumination (Germer and Neff, 2017). These reactions are the opposite of self-compassion.

In mindfulness, we are bringing awareness to our experience—the body sensations, thoughts, and emotions. With self-compassion, we are bringing awareness to the one having the experience. Both are needed in order to change your relationship with suffering. And you may find that both are also helpful in changing your relationship to yourself.

SELF-COMPASSION BREAK

To bring this into action, let's try another practice adapted from the *Mindful Self-Compassion*

Workbook (Neff and Germer, 2018). It's called the "self-compassion break." Try it now in a formal way, but be aware that this is a practice that can be done at any time and anywhere more informally, whenever you are experiencing difficulty. When you notice that you are feeling frustration, grief, or fear about your sleep, try meeting the experience this way:

- Bring to mind the thoughts and emotions you have about not being able to sleep in the way that you may be used to or want to. Allow yourself to really get in touch with all the longings for what you want your sleep to look like, and with the resistance to what your sleep looks like now.

- Allow yourself to really feel what these feelings feel like in your body. Try to notice where you might feel them most strongly.

- Acknowledge kindly to yourself: *"This is a moment of suffering."* You could also say to yourself, *"Ouch, this hurts!"* or, *"This is hard to bear."*

- Breathe in and out and allow this experience and your feelings to be exactly as they are.

- Next, remind yourself that *suffering is part of the human experience* and that you are not alone. Actually say to yourself, *"I am not alone"* or, *"Other people experience this too."*

- Breathe in and out and remind yourself of the truth of your common humanity.

- Now, place your hand or both of your hands over your heart. Feel the warmth and presence of your own hand and let that gesture of comfort stream into you.

- Say to yourself, *"May I be kind to myself."* Remember that when anyone (including you) is suffering, kindness and care are what is needed. Other words of comfort you can try are: *"May I give myself the compassion that I need," "May I forgive myself for being human," "I care about you and am right here."* Anything that you might say to a good friend, try saying to yourself.

- Breathe in and out and extend warmth and kindness to this one who is suffering. This one who is called *you.*

Like all of the practices that we are offering in this book, this is not a "trick" to stop your feelings. A fundamental message in mindful self-compassion is that we don't give ourselves compassion to fix or even transform suffering. We give ourselves compassion because we *are* suffering. It's that simple. You, too, are a being who experiences the tenderness of the human condition. You, too, feel weak, frustrated, and powerless sometimes. You are just as deserving of compassion as anyone else.

Many people struggle with that realization. They think, "I just need to tough it out," or "If I give myself compassion, then I'm just giving in to self-pity and being a wimp." But let's look at it this way. Self-pity lacks the perspective that others suffer too; it's absorbed in the drama of its own story. Self-compassion, on the other hand, acknowledges that all people suffer. It creates a container of awareness in which to experience suffering without making any additional stories about it. Research shows that people who are compassionate toward themselves are actually much more likely to have an accurate appraisal of themselves and their faults without going into shame. They are therefore able to recover more quickly from difficult experiences and to bounce back and access the resources they need to support them. This is what self-compassion has to offer you, too.

So, as you continue to practice the GMATI meditations as well as any of the other meditations, try bringing in some self-compassion to support your practice. Additionally, try making the self-compassion break a routine practice whenever you notice yourself struggling with any kind of discomfort. Like planting seeds in a garden, you just may find that if you plant self-compassion in your life and nurture it daily, you will become more at ease and resilient in how you feel about yourself and how you deal with the stresses of insomnia.

Bearing in mind this possibility of befriending yourself with compassion, it's now time to practice the GMATI-2 meditation again.

***

When you have finished the meditation, take a few minutes to write in your journal. Remembering that nonjudgment is at the heart of mindfulness, what did you notice:

- In your body?

- In your mind?

- And in your mood?

Day 7: The Stability of a Mountain

It's the last day of your second week of practicing GMATI! You are certainly gaining traction and hopefully settling in to the routine of a daily mindfulness practice.

You may also be noticing that you periodically feel bombarded by all the thoughts, feelings, and changing body sensations you experience during meditation. So today, we're going to suggest some additional ways you can cultivate a sense of stability in the midst of changing experiences while you are practicing the GMATI-2 meditation. We invite you to use some imagery, along with an intention to bring certain qualities into your posture and your meditation experience. For many people, imagery can invoke a quality of feeling that can be of great benefit in dealing with the experience of tension that comes from the resistance to insomnia.

But for some people, creating images in the mind is not so easy. If this is true for you, don't worry. The sophistication of the image is less important than the intention. The more we understand the brain, the more we can know about the effects of particular mental activities like mentally creating imagery. When athletes use guided imagery to just imagine themselves engaging in their sport, the same regions of the brain light up (become activated) that correspond to the muscles and body systems required for the sport (Clarey, 2014; Barraclough). It's as if the brain doesn't really know that all the athlete is doing at that moment is just sitting in his or her room imagining. And something great about this absorbed focus in the brain is that if it is busy with the guided imagery, it can't be busy reacting to the deleterious effects of insomnia.

In his book *Wherever You Go, There You Are: Mindfulness Meditation in Everyday Life* (1994, pp.135-140), Jon Kabat-Zinn introduced this way of using the imagery of a mountain to support meditation practice:

THE IMAGE OF A MOUNTAIN

Try picturing in your mind's eye, as best you can, the most beautiful mountain that you know. Maybe it's one that you have seen, or even climbed. Or just one that you create in your imagination right now. Allow the image and even the *feeling* of this mountain to come gradually into greater and greater focus.

See if you can engage all your senses to fully experience this mountain in your mind. What do you notice about its overall shape? Does it have one lofty peak that rises high into the sky? Or is there a series of peaks? See if you can imagine the large base of the mountain that is rooted in the rock of the earth's crust. Picture its either steep or gently sloping sides. Take time to notice and to feel how massive it is, how solid, how unmoving, how beautiful—both from afar and up close. All the way from the top, stretching majestically to the sky, down to the massive base that anchors the mountain into the earth. See the whole mountain in front of you; the top, the base, and the sides of the mountain. Really notice how steady, solid, and beautiful it is.

Merge with the Feeling of the Mountain

Now, see if you can bring the sense of mountain into your own body, so that your body sitting here and the mountain that you have just created in your mind's eye become one. Start to feel that as you sit here, you begin to share in the massiveness and the stillness and the majesty of your mountain. You become the mountain—rooted in your own sitting posture. Your head becomes the lofty peak, which is supported by the rest of your body and is affording you a panoramic vista. Your shoulders and arms are the sides of the mountain. Your buttocks and legs are the solid base, rooted to and rising up from your seat. Experience in your body a sense of uplift from deep within your pelvis and spine.

Now take a moment to pay attention to your breath; with each breath, you are becoming a little more of a breathing mountain. Breathing in this way, you can be steadfast in your stillness. You are completely what you are, beyond the thoughts or feelings that swirl through your mind. Like a mountain, you are in this moment a centered, rooted, unmoving presence.

The Mountain Is Unwavering through All Changes

Continuing with your imagination, become aware of what happens as the sun travels across the sky. See the light and shadows and colors and how they are changing virtually moment by moment across the mountain's granite stillness. You can imagine and feel how night follows day, and day follows night. One flowing into the next. There might be a canopy of stars, the moon, and then the sun once again.

Through it all, the mountain just sits, experiencing change in each and every moment.

On the surface, the mountain is constantly changing, and yet underneath, it is always just being itself. It remains still as the weather changes moment by moment, day by day, and seasons flow from one to another. The mountain exudes a calmness and it abides through all change. In summer, there may be no snow on the mountain, except perhaps for the tallest peaks or in bluffs that are shielded from direct sunlight. In the fall, the mountain may wear a coat of brilliant colors. In winter, it is blanketed in snow and ice. In any season it may find itself at times enshrouded in clouds or fog, or pummeled by bitter rains. At times, the mountain may be visited by violent storms, buffeted by snow and rain and winds. Throughout all these changes, feel the solid stillness of the mountain as the solid stillness of your own being, as you continue to sit, continuing to be a "breathing mountain."

The Mountain Experiences Renewal and Outward Changes

With the inevitable changing of seasons, spring comes, and with it, the birds sing in the trees once again. Leaves return and flowers start to bloom in the high meadows and on the slopes. Trickling streams start to overflow with the melting snow. Through it all, the mountain continues to sit. It is still unmoved by the weather and by what is happening on the surface. It is not shaken by the world of appearances.

The Mountain Does Not Concern Itself with the Opinion of Others

Now, imagine what happens as people visit the mountain. They may comment on how beautiful it is, or they may complain how "it's not a good day to see the mountain," that "it's too cloudy or rainy or foggy or dark." None of this matters to the mountain. It remains at all times its essential self, unconcerned with opinions. It knows that clouds may come and clouds may go. People may like it or they may not. The mountain's magnificence and beauty are not changed one bit by whether people see it or not, or by the weather. Whether it is seen or unseen, enveloped in sun or clouds, experiencing broiling or frigid temperatures, going through day or night, it just sits, calmly being itself.

Finding Peace and Stillness through All Kinds of Change

In the same way as we sit in meditation, we can experience and become the "mountain." We can embody the same unwavering stillness and rootedness in the face of everything that changes in our own lives—the changes that occur over seconds and minutes, which turn into hours and then years. Jon

Kabat-Zinn (1994, p.139) reminds us: "In our lives and in our meditation practice, we experience constantly the changing nature of mind and body and of the outer world. We experience periods of light and dark, vivid color and drab dullness. We experience storms of varying intensity and violence, in the outer world and in our own lives and minds. Buffeted by high winds, by cold and rain, we endure periods of darkness and pain as well as savoring moments of joy and uplift. Even our appearance changes constantly, experiencing a weathering of its own."

EXPERIENCING EQUANIMITY

By developing the image of this mountain in your meditation practice, you can borrow its strength and stability and take it in as your own. You may even gain support from the inner qualities of the mountain to face each moment of your meditation, your struggle with insomnia, and in fact the rest of your life, with a kind of equanimity. Perhaps then, just like the varying natural experiences—seasons, storms, and weather patterns that happen to the mountain, you can come to experience the constant changes and fluctuations that happen in your own life, and in your own mind and heart, as a kind of "weather." Jon again says, "We tend to take it all personally. But its strongest characteristic is impersonal. The weather of our own lives is not to be ignored or denied. It is to be encountered, honored, felt, known for what it is, and held in awareness. And in holding it in this way, we come to know a deeper silence and stillness and wisdom. Mountains have this to teach us and much more if we can come to listen."

So, see how it is to use this mountain imagery from time to time as you practice the GMATI meditations. See if it can remind you of what it feels like to sit mindfully with a sense of resolve and stillness.

If you want to practice a guided version of the Mountain Meditation, you can find a recording of it on the New Harbinger website (http://www.newharbinger.com/42587). But for now, just experiment with being the mountain in your imagination as you now practice the GMATI-2 meditation.

**

Now, remembering that nonjudgment is at the heart of mindfulness, what did you notice as you meditated:

- In your body?

- In your mind?

- And in your mood?

You have now completed half of the GMATI series and are probably beginning to notice changes in your relationship to your sleep and the emotions that accompany it. There is more to come that will take you even further. Stay with it and reap the rewards!

CHAPTER 6

GMATI—Week 3

In Week 1, we looked at how the struggle with sleepiness worsens insomnia. We then discussed how mindfulness meditation can help with this struggle, and to that end, you practiced the first GMATI meditation. You also explored ways to cultivate "awareness" by bringing moments of pause into your day and doing daily activities as a meditation.

In Week 2, we emphasized how mindfulness meditation can help you to *accept* your sleep as it is and in this way, help break the vicious cycle of trying unsuccessfully to control insomnia—which only leads to increased arousal and even worse sleep. We guided you through a body scan meditation emphasizing acceptance, and explored how to experience sensations in the body, including the sensations of release through some mindful stretching. We introduced you to ways in which bringing compassion to yourself can also help you navigate the challenges of insomnia.

We've done a lot so far, but there is more to how mindfulness can help you experience less suffering related to insomnia. The theme we'll be focused on here in Week 3 is "letting go."

When we start paying attention to our inner experience, we rapidly discover that there are certain thoughts and feelings that the mind seems to want to hold on to. Similarly, there are many thoughts and feelings that we try to get rid of or to avoid experiencing, because they are unpleasant or painful or frightening.

In our meditation practice, we intentionally put aside the tendency to elevate some aspects of our experience and to reject others. Instead, we just let our experience be what it is and practice observing it from moment to moment. Letting go is a way of letting things be, of accepting things as they are. When we observe our own mind grasping and pushing away, we remind ourselves to purposefully let go of those impulses, just to see what will happen if we do. When we find ourselves judging our experience, we let go of those judging thoughts. When thoughts of the past or of the future come up, we let go of those as well. We just watch.

Letting go means releasing something—you could also try "letting be" as an easier preliminary step in that direction. Imagine you were holding on to a small stone. If you let it go, you have to turn your hand to face downward and open your fingers, which are grasping the stone, in order for it to "go" from you. If you "let it be," you are simply letting it rest in the palm of your hand. It's just there. You're not holding on to it, or actively trying to get rid of it. It's another facet of acceptance. From here, you can bring curiosity into it, or expand your attention around whatever it is you are letting be, and see what else is part of your experience of the present moment.

As in previous weeks, we encourage you to first read through this week's new meditation so that you become familiar with the instructions and begin to mentally "download" the kind of guidance that supports the experience of "letting go." But remember, reading is not the same thing as practicing! You need to actually listen to the recording and practice it daily to fully "exercise" this learning.

GMATI-3 MEDITATION

Once you are in a comfortable position, connect with an intention that will support your practice. It could be something like "I'm taking this time to be with myself and allow myself and this moment to be exactly as they are."

Start by taking a few moments to welcome yourself into this time and place—switching from a mode of doing this and doing that, planning for the future and rehashing the past, into a mode of simple being. Of just being in the present moment, just as it is, knowing there is no place to go right now, nothing to do. Releasing all effort for doing, all trying. Allowing yourself to just be aware of being right here and right now. Opening to the experience of sensing directly what is present, with no need to try to analyze or problem solve. It may be helpful to think of this as a time for you. A time to simply be with yourself, a time of just letting be.

Begin to notice all the places that your body is in contact with something solid. It could be the chair under your seat, the ground against your legs or feet, your hands resting in your lap. Allow yourself to feel these sensations of contact and enable the body to know that in this very moment, it is being held and supported, and that it is safe. Gravity is holding you in place. You don't need to work too hard to be sitting here, and so you can ease into the support and allow your weight to rest on what is holding you.

In addition to the sensations of contact with solid surfaces, see if you can also feel how your body is in contact with space. Maybe you notice the passage of air against your skin, or the feeling of temperature. Feel where you end and the space around you begins.

Now, notice that without your having to do anything in particular, you are breathing. Simply become aware of the sensations of the breath as it enters the body and as it leaves the body. Perhaps noticing the subtle movements in your abdomen as you breathe in and out—how the belly expands on the inhalation, and then softens on the exhalation. No need to control it. Simply breathe normally and breathe naturally, moment to moment, controlling only your awareness. Breathing is all there is.

When you notice that the mind has wandered, gently congratulate yourself for being aware of this experience. You may also notice thoughts about the thoughts. The mind may even label thoughts and emotions with evaluations such as "bad" or "getting worse." If so, just gently and compassionately acknowledge wherever the mind has wandered. Accept the thoughts just as they are. And then, gently escort yourself back to an awareness of the body breathing—the breath coming in and the breath going out.

Now, imagine that you are standing on the edge of a train platform. Imagine your thoughts as trains, going by the station one at a time. Observe each thought, whatever comes to mind, and inwardly note to yourself "thought" or "thinking." There are no right thoughts or wrong thoughts; some might be fast-moving and some might be slower, lumbering ones. Rather than focusing on the thought and thinking about where it will lead (for example, getting on the train), stand back and just observe the thought. If you have stepped on a train, gently bring yourself back to the platform and return to simply observing the train. Bringing your attention back to the breath is like coming back to the "platform." Just notice the breathing in and the breathing out.

As best you can, also bring an attitude of generous allowance and gentle acceptance to your experience. There is nothing to be fixed, no particular state to be achieved. Simply allow the experience to be your experience, with no need to be other than what it is.

Now, move your attention from the sensations of breath and bring it to the sensations of the body as a whole. Feeling how the whole body is connected. Just noticing, just being with the body. No need to get involved in liking or disliking what we are aware of in our body. Just accepting what simply exists and letting be. Just noticing the changing nature of the bodily sensations—how they come and go. Simply being mindful of sensations rising and passing. Feeling the head connected to the neck. Feeling the connection of the neck to the shoulders, arms, and hands, then moving on to how the arms are connected to the chest, then on to the back, and to the belly. Now noticing the hips, legs, feet. Feeling the body as a whole organism with simple awareness.

Don't try to hold on to body sensations or make them go away. Just let them be. Just let them come and go as they will.

Now, gently expand your awareness from the body and turn your attention to any emotions or thoughts that may be present right now. Just accepting them as they are. Noticing that like body sensations, even thoughts and emotions can come and go—they too are often changing. Include the thinking and the feeling as a part of your practice of simply being aware of what is arising. Acknowledge their presence, accepting them, then letting them go.

Also make room for any tensions or anxieties. Just allow them to be there. Watch how these emotions change from moment to moment—sometimes growing stronger, sometimes growing weaker, and sometimes staying the same. It does not matter; just let them be.

The intention is not to make you feel better, but to get better at feeling and allowing feeling.

Now, bring to mind any feelings or thoughts specifically about your difficulties with sleep. Shift your awareness toward the discomfort you have with your sleep. See if you can shine the light of your awareness on it, even if the discomfort is strong. Allow yourself to be present with your fears and anxieties about your sleep. Start with "recognizing" what is here.

Notice if what you are experiencing are doubts, worries, reservations, or something else. You can even inwardly note them to yourself, silently acknowledging "doubt," "fear," "frustration," "grief," or whatever it is you are finding.

Then, practice just allowing them to be exactly as they are. There is no need to try and work on them or change them. Simply be aware and accepting. You can even mentally whisper an encouraging and soothing word or phrase to yourself. Something like "Let it be," or "It's okay to feel this." Gently relax the edges of your resistance.

Stay as long as possible with this discomfort and try to breathe into and around it. Just like you would with an area of tension or discomfort in the body.

Have the intention to accept it and allow it to be, while bringing focused and compassionate attention to the sensations of discomfort.

If you notice yourself tensing up and resisting or pushing away from the experience, acknowledge this and see if you can make space for this experience too.

This thought or feeling is not necessarily your enemy. Just notice it and let it be. Just let it be your experience right now.

If sensations of discomfort grow stronger, you can acknowledge their presence, perhaps staying with them, breathing into them, and accepting them.

You may also notice thoughts about your discomfort, or even thoughts about your thoughts. If so, it is okay; just let them be. Let them come and go on their own.

You may notice your mind coming up with evaluative labels, such as "bad" or "getting worse." If so, thank your mind for the label and return to just the experience as you let go of the label.

If you become overwhelmed by the thoughts and feelings arising, you can always come back to the sensations of the body in contact with whatever you are sitting on, or to the breath, to ground yourself and be in a place of refuge until you are ready to turn toward the discomfort once again.

Notice the tendency of the mind to start telling stories about this discomfort or to predicting the future. If this happens, you can go back to just observing these narratives as thoughts—or like a full train passing by. And then reopen your attention to the direct experience of the difficulty in your body. What it feels like, rather than whatever narrative the mind tells about it.

Allow yourself to stay with your discomfort for as long as it pulls on your attention. When you discover anxiety and discomfort are no longer pulling for your attention, then let them go.

Now, gently withdraw from any thoughts, discomfort, or anxiety, coming back to feeling the body as a whole. Feeling yourself connected from head to toe and to fingertips; feeling the whole body resting in this seated posture you are in. Feeling the whole body breathing.

Take these last few moments to feel some gratitude toward yourself for having made this effort for your health and well-being. For having taken time to simply be present with your experience as it is without the need to make it any different. For simply accepting what you are aware of. For allowing what you are aware of to come and then go without the need to do anything. To simply be present.

Now, bring some small movements back into the body. Stretch fingers and toes, hands and feet, neck, or anything else that needs stretching. Recognizing that this feeling of presence, of focus, that you have just experienced is as close as the next moment—as close as the next breath.

Day 1: Working with Thoughts

In order to truly understand what it means to "let go," we need to spend a little time exploring how much thoughts influence what you are experiencing in the present moment. Many people who start practicing meditation believe they need to "clear their mind of thoughts" in order to experience the relief of "letting go." But letting go is different than clearing your mind or forcing thoughts to go away. Like many people, you may have tried pushing your thoughts away, only to find that the thoughts keep coming back. They may even get stronger in the process. In contrast, letting go is a way of mindfully being *aware* of your thoughts, letting them be as they are without judging or evaluating them, and then allowing them to dissolve back into the ether from which they sprang. You will find that if you let these thoughts come in and go out of your conscious awareness without getting engaged in them, they will eventually subside.

This is a very different and maybe even counterintuitive way to approach thoughts that you wished you didn't have in the first place! Trying to push them away or to clear your mind is usually nearly impossible. The mind thinks. That's what it does! On the other hand, our thoughts tend to successively come and then go if we let them. Let's try a little exercise to become more aware of this.

NOTICING THE THINKER

- Close your eyes for about sixty seconds and just be mindful of any thoughts or images that bubble up into your mind.

- As soon as you experience a thought or image, say softly to yourself the word "thought," or just give it a number (one, two, three...) and starting counting them as they arise. Then, gently return your attention back to noticing if and when any more arise.

- If no thoughts turn up, which can sometimes happen, you may find yourself thinking that "*no thoughts appear to be arriving,*" which in itself is a thought. So go ahead label that one "*thought*" too.

- After about a minute, check in—how many thoughts did you notice? The number of them doesn't matter in the least. What's important here is that you are actually observing thoughts.

- Did you notice how the thoughts come and then go?

Thoughts do come and go, but forcing them to go in one direction is like trying to reverse the flow of a powerful river. We are suggesting that you see what happens when you just let your thoughts about your sleep run their course; let them come and then go. Rather than trying to block or reverse the flow of this river of thoughts, think of standing on the bank of this river observing it as it goes by and letting go of the effort of trying to force these thoughts to go in a certain direction. Mindfulness can show you how you can let go of your thoughts about your sleep problems, without getting caught up in them.

Some would ask, "Isn't this just giving up and giving in to poor sleep?" No, this is not passively giving in; this is not resignation. It is actually quite the opposite! Rather than giving up, you are making a conscious decision to accept or even embrace what is happening, and then just letting it go. You are choosing to actively respond by allowing thoughts and feelings to just be, rather than automatically avoiding, reacting to, or trying desperately to change the unpleasant feeling or experience. In this way, you might even find that the experience itself changes—that the negative emotions really were not as bad as you thought.

For example, rather than always worrying about how badly you slept the night before, or how bad tomorrow will be if you have another poor night of sleep, just try to be mindfully aware of these thoughts. When you simply notice these thoughts, you can accept them and then let them go and no longer be caught up in them. When people with insomnia realize that they can stop struggling, they often describe feeling lighter and more able to float with their problems, rather than being pulled under by them.

If you have ever blown bubbles, you have a good reference for what is actually happening with all that thinking. A bubble is blown. You can see it. It has a form, a shape, and maybe even a sheen or color to it. You may even be able to lightly touch it, but then—pop. It's not there anymore. This is exactly how it is with thoughts. They have no more substance as distinct things than bubbles.

So as you experiment with accepting the thoughts that show up and then letting them go, try remembering their "bubblelike" nature. Acceptance and letting go are important steps for you to take. They will help set you on the path toward improving your insomnia, leading to less struggle and arousal, improved sleep quality, and energy conservation, resulting in an enhanced quality of life. In this way, you can even start to reestablish a positive association between your sleep and your bed. By promoting a healthy and flexible approach to sleep, any negative associations (and therefore arousal levels) will be reduced, creating a platform from which natural sleep can emerge effortlessly.

With the GMATI series and all the other supportive mindfulness and self-compassion practices, you can let go of all your thoughts about your sleep problems.

And now it's time to practice the GMATI-3 meditation.

***

When you are through, take out your journal and notice how it was to relate to thoughts in this way.

Remembering that nonjudgment is at the heart of mindfulness, take some time with your journal and ask yourself: What did you notice:

- In your body?

- In your mind?

- And in your mood?

Day 2: Befriending Emotions

You're on to your second day of practicing turning toward any difficult thoughts or emotions specifically related to your insomnia while you're meditating. We know this can be hard, so it's incredibly important that you be patient and respectful toward yourself as you attempt to do this. Difficult emotions such as anxiety, fear, sadness, and despair cause you to feel pain. When you turn toward these kinds of experiences, even with mindfulness and compassion, that pain may temporarily increase.

Many people who attempt to do this in meditation often wonder, "Well, just how much pain or distress should I allow into my meditation practice?" The answer, according to Zen Master and Vietnamese meditation teacher Thich Nhat Hanh, is: "Not much!"

While it's true that experiencing discomfort is necessary to enable self-compassion to arise and for emotions to be more skillfully worked through, you only actually need to "touch" it just a little bit. You don't need to flood yourself with intense emotion, because that would just overwhelm you and could start to "hardwire" those emotions even more, which is the complete opposite of what you're trying to do.

The skillful way of opening to strong emotions is to *gradually* incline toward the difficulty with mindfulness and self-compassion. The mindful self-compassion program identifies stages to doing this. These stages are helpful to identify and get familiar with on your path to "acceptance" and "letting go." They are just like what you might imagine the various stages are of how you encounter strangers at your home. Since *resistance* is so well conditioned into the human experience, we often tend to start there. When we are in resistance, we may block the door and yell at the "visitors" to "go away!" You may also do this because you are taken off guard and are reacting to the experience, and don't really know what's there. But once you move past resistance, what comes next in each successive stage is a gradual release of emotional opposition that we could call "letting go." See if these stages ring true for you.

Curiosity

Just like in all mindfulness practices, bringing in an attitude of curiosity allows you to begin exploring what is there. It's like peeping through the peep hole.

Tolerating

Here, you are starting to safely endure what you notice. Like asking the guests to stay just on the threshold or in the foyer of the house, you are holding steady where you are.

Allowing

With allowing, you are letting the feelings come and go. Now you are allowing the guests into your house to look around.

Befriending

Here, you have grown accustomed to their presence, and may even sit down to listen to what they have to say. With emotions, you are seeing the value in all human experiences, including difficulty. You are open and understanding of the complex and rich tapestry of emotions that flesh out each human life.

This process of learning to turn toward and befriend your inner experience is not new. The fourteenth-century Sufi mystic Rumi wrote in his famous poem "The Guesthouse":

This being human is a guest house.
Every morning a new arrival.
A joy, a depression, a meanness,
some momentary awareness comes
as an unexpected visitor.
Welcome and entertain them all!

This six-hundred-year-old poem has something to teach us, or at least inspire us to reflect on, as we learn to be with the myriad emotions that show up from day to day, from moment to moment. What would it really be like to "welcome and entertain them all"? Perhaps these "guests" have something to offer. About their inherently impermanent nature, but also about your own ability to feel what you feel with wisdom and kindness.

Labeling Emotions

In the meditation this week, we also gave you prompts for labeling whatever emotions you are finding, asking yourself with curiosity, "What is this emotion?" There is a saying that you "name it to tame it." When you actually name what emotion is present, you start to become less fused to it. It gets a little less sticky and you have some space around the feeling in which to engage it.

Psychological and neuroscience researcher David Creswell and his colleagues (Creswell et al., 2007) found that when you label difficult emotions, the activity in the amygdala (which is the part of the brain we talked about in chapter 1 that is responsible for registering danger) becomes less active and less likely to trigger a stress reaction in the body. But how you label the emotions is super important! It's very important to bring in a gentle and accepting tone to your labeling.

The next step in working with emotions is to move your awareness of the emotion into how it actually feels in the body, because an emotion is a combination of thoughts and body sensations. Frustration, for example, may show up in the mind as thoughts about how "you are not getting what you want or need in the moment" and "what you should have said or shouldn't have said to anyone who may have been involved." But it also includes some kinds of tensions in the body, perhaps in the chest, throat, or abdomen. You may even feel an increase of heat, or perhaps a cool numbness, somewhere in the body.

Now, it's a lot trickier to try to manage difficult emotions by focusing only on thoughts. Thoughts are "slippery" and quickly move from one to another. When you stay in the realm of the thoughts related to an emotion, you end up telling yourself more and more stories about why you are frustrated, and then the emotion of frustration increases rather than decreases. But the way emotions show up in the body is a bit slower moving and easier to pay attention to without adding so much fuel to the fire. So you locate the emotion in the body and then anchor your attention there with kindness and affection.

With this kind of loving and accepting relationship to the emotion, you see that it is not as solid as it may have seemed, and it begins to change all on its own. When your awareness has a fearful or disdainful quality to it, you will be less likely to open to it. But if you are tending to it in a warm and tender way, you have the strength to feel it and to be present for whatever is happening with it. You "let go" of needing it to be different.

Once you've named the emotion and felt it in the body, try the following ways to support yourself in being with it (Neff and Germer, 2018):

- *Softening:* Allow yourself to soften into the location in the body where you are experiencing the emotion. Let all your muscles soften and relax, as if you were slipping either your whole body or just this area of the body into a nice warm bath. You can even say to yourself—*softening, softening, softening.*

- *Soothing:* Try placing a hand over your heart or right on the place in the body that feels uncomfortable and open to the warmth and tenderness streaming into your body from your hand. You can imagine it as if you were breathing right into this area—as if your breath were tenderly touching the discomfort from the inside. You can even add some words of comfort to yourself, such as "It's okay, I can feel this even though it's hard," or "May I be kind to myself." Knowing that you can always come back to your breath if it begins to feel too strong. Otherwise, staying with it and maybe repeating—*soothing, soothing, soothing.*

- *Allowing:* Just make room for the discomfort to be there and release the need to make it go away. This is *letting go.* You are letting go of the need to be any different from how you are. Repeating to yourself *allowing, allowing, allowing.*

Now, with this in mind, it's time to practice the GMATI-3 meditation. Bring in an attitude of curiosity and maybe even of allowing while you do the practice.

***

When you have finished, take a few moments to note in your journal:

- What did you notice when you labeled the emotion?

- What happened when you became aware of the emotion in the body?

- What else did you notice in your body overall, in your thoughts and with your emotions?

Day 3: Letting Go into Stretching

Thoughts and emotions and body sensations, oh my! Today, we'll go back to doing some stretching to help with all this awareness. Try doing this practice lying down on the floor. We'll be paying extra attention to the physical experience of "letting go." (You can find a recording for this practice on the New Harbinger website: http://www.newharbinger.com/42587.)

You may even want to try practicing the GMATI-3 meditation today from this position of lying on the floor after going through the stretching. If so, make sure you have whatever you are using to listen to the guidance right nearby, so you don't have to get up to start the practice.

Start by lying on your back on a mat on the floor. Let your feet be uncrossed and rest your arms alongside your body. Take a few deep breaths to help yourself connect to the flow of breathing, releasing into the support of the floor. Know that you can always come back to the feeling of the breath if something in the guidance doesn't feel appropriate for your body, or if you just need to stabilize your attention.

1. Now, slowly allow your arms to start to rise up off the floor and reach up toward the ceiling and then toward the wall beyond your head. From here, stretch the full length of your body, from your hands to your feet. And then, slowly let your arms come back down to rest alongside your body once again. Feel the wash of release that happens when the stretch is finished

2. Bend both of your knees and let your feet rest on the floor about hips-width distance apart. Start to tip your pelvis so that the small arc in the

lower back presses into the floor. Now, rock the pelvis in the opposite direction so that you accentuate the curve in your lumbar spine. Slowly rock the pelvis back and forth, moving between these two positions to create some release in your lower back.

3.   Draw your knees toward your chest and use your arms to hug your legs in toward you. Allow your body to rock back and forth and from side to side.

4.   Now, hug your legs even tighter, giving yourself a real squeeze. Become a small little ball and then release your arms and legs and settle back into your beginning resting pose.

5.   Bend your knees once again and place your feet on the floor. Draw one knee in toward your chest and then let the other leg stretch back down onto the floor. You can even let your head come off the floor and bring your nose toward your knee to increase the stretch. Now, switch to the other leg so that you get a stretch on the opposite side. When you have stretched both legs, come back to your original resting pose and just feel what sensations are present in your body.

6.   Once again, come back to the knees-bent, feet-on-the-floor position. Now, lift one foot up toward the ceiling so the leg is stretching upward and you feel some activation in the back of your leg. Take hold of your leg with your hands. You can

hold on to your leg behind the thigh, knee, or calf, depending on the level of flexibility in your hamstrings. Just let yourself feel the sensations of stretching that are likely happening at the back of your leg. You can try softening, soothing, and allowing with the sensations. You can also try directing your breath into the sensations of stretch. Just hanging out right at the edge of the stretch—not pushing past what is wise for you, so that there is pain, but not staying so far away from the stretch that there are no sensations. After a little time of just allowing and "letting go," you may find a change in your flexibility. Once you've experienced some ease in the stretch, allow the leg to slowly float back down toward the floor. Once it arrives, feel the wash of release that happens after the stretch. Now repeat this on the other side.

7. Now, roll over and bring yourself onto your hands and knees into a kind of tabletop position. Let your chest and belly sag toward the floor like the sagging back of a cow while letting the back of your head incline back toward your tailbone. Then, reverse and let your back arch up toward the ceiling, like a cat arching its back, and let your head drop down. Go back and forth between "cow" and "cat" poses to bring fluid stretching movement into the spine.

8. Roll back down onto your back and allow yourself to rest for a moment. Then draw your knees in

toward your chest, and then allow your arms to reach out to the sides into a T position, with your hands resting downward on the floor. Let your knees gently fall toward the floor on one side while keeping your arms in a relaxed T. Experience the gentle twist in your spine and breathe into the sensations in your back. Then, let your legs fall to the opposite side and experience the twist there. Now, draw your knees back in toward your chest and give them a squeeze again.

9. Let your legs and arms come back into the rest pose, just lying on the floor.

It's time to begin the GMATI-3 meditation, if you haven't done so already.

***

When you are finished with the meditation, take some time for reflection in your journal, noticing what you experienced in your body as "letting go." Now, remembering that nonjudgment is at the heart of mindfulness, what did you notice:

• In your body?

• In your mind?

• And in your mood?

Day 4: The Practice of RAIN

The theme this week is "letting go," but as you may have noticed, this can be easier said than done. Most of us human beings have done a great job at conditioning ourselves to do the exact opposite. Instead of "letting go," we resist, cling to, or avoid whatever is happening in the present moment. We do this sometimes by lashing out, having a cigarette, bingeing on Netflix, scrolling through Facebook, or getting immersed in obsessive thinking. All of these attempts to control life and what we might be feeling within can actually cut us off from feeling alive and in connection with our hearts.

This reaction is very likely when you are sick and tired about your insomnia.

We need ways to come back to our hearts when we are feeling overwhelmed and out of control. So, to give you some really rich tools, we're going to be combining the "softening, soothing, allowing" procedure from the mindful self-compassion program with a practice called RAIN, which was developed by a group of meditation teachers and popularized by Tara Brach in her book *True Refuge: Finding Peace and Freedom in Your Own Awakened Heart* (2013).

Here are the steps of RAIN:

R—Recognize what is happening.
A—Allow life to be just as it is.

I—Investigate inner experience with kindness.
N—Non-identification.

Recognize What Is Happening

We begin by opening to what is actually happening within us in the present moment. When you shine the light of your attention on whatever thoughts, emotions, feelings, or sensations are arising right here and now, you can recognize and know that that is what's present. However, you may have already noticed that some parts of your present-moment experience are easier to connect with than others.

If someone were to ask you "How are you?" you might say: "Anxious." That's usually because you're aware of the thoughts that are running through the mind. It might be a new experience to for you to open to the actual sensations of a squeezing, pressure, or tightness occurring in the body that accompany anxiety. On the other hand, if physical sensations are very strong and you're experiencing jittery nervousness or tightness in the chest or shallow breathing, *that* may be where your attention immediately goes. You may not be aware of the underlying thoughts or beliefs that are triggering the jitteriness—thoughts like "I can't do this!" or "What if I fail?" But when you pause and ask yourself: "What is happening inside me right now?" you can awaken recognition. Remember that having a friendly and curious attitude toward yourself and your experiences can help you uncover whatever is there and let go of judging yourself for it.

Allow Life to Be Just as It Is

To really open and allow, we sometimes first need to experience a kind of softening around what is hurting. You can do this by doing the "softening, soothing, allowing" procedure we introduced you to in day 2. Start by letting all your muscles soften and relax. You can even say to yourself—*softening, softening, softening.*

Then, you can focus on soothing yourself as you're experiencing the discomfort, and maybe repeating—*soothing, soothing, soothing.*

Then, you can connect with your intention to "allow." Just make room for the discomfort to be there and release the need to make it go away, while repeating to yourself—*allowing, allowing, allowing.* This is letting go.

Just a reminder that "allowing" means letting the thoughts, emotions, feelings, or sensations you discover to be exactly as they are, at least for these few moments. It's perfectly natural to feel resistant to what you are experiencing and to just wish the whole thing would "go away." So this is a practice where you can allow those thoughts and feelings to just be there too. You don't even need to fix or change your aversion.

You are supporting your resolve to "let be" or "let go" when you mentally whisper an encouraging word or phrase to yourself. Some other supportive words you can use now are "Yes, this too," or "I consent." Saying yes to yourself no matter what has arisen, whether it be fear, frustration, grief, or anything else, allows the sharp edges of the pain to soften. It's not that you are saying "Yes, I will always have insomnia," or "I will never sleep again." You are simply consenting to what is already happening in the present moment and offering it no resistance. Tara Brach says about this part of the practice that when you "offer the phrase gently and patiently ... in time, your defenses will relax, and you may feel a physical sense of yielding or opening to waves of experience" (2013).

Investigate with Kindness

The first two steps of RAIN can at times be enough to provide relief and reconnect you with presence. But these next two steps are helpful when you are triggered over and over to experience the same overwhelming feelings. In fact, each night, as you anticipate going to bed, you may be anxious about what will happen and how it will likely be another sleepless night. These kinds of repetitive experiences of pain are more deeply understood by strengthening mindful awareness through this particular kind of *investigation,* which is the "I" of RAIN.

Investigation means calling on the attitude of curiosity that is fundamental to the cultivation of mindfulness. With curiosity, we move in close to see the truth of what's here. The first step of investigation is to recognize what is happening in the present moment—both outside and inside of you. But now, you engage in an even more active and pointed inquiry. You might ask yourself: "What most wants attention right now?" "How am I experiencing this in my body?" "What am I believing?" or "What does this feeling want from me?" Again, Tara Brach teaches: "You might contact sensations of hollowness or shakiness, and then find a sense of unworthiness and shame buried in these feelings. Unless they are brought into consciousness, these beliefs and emotions will control your experience and perpetuate your identification with a limited, deficient self" (2018).

Now, at this point in the investigation, you need to be really wise. It's very normal that when you try to investigate something, it just stimulates judgments about the feeling or the impulse to find immediate relief, so that you can solve the problem and make it go away. No one wants to feel uncomfortable, and so it's perfectly natural that resistance will arise. As we've said before, resistance can come in the form of lots of thoughts (and judgments) swimming around in your head, leaving you bereft of the feeling of presence within the body. So what is needed here is *lots* of kindness.

Imagine that your child or a dear friend came to you after a day of being harassed and bullied. If you met her with judgment or a must-fixit attitude, you are unlikely to get at what really happened and what she might be feeling, leaving her no better off. But if you meet her with warmth, kindness, and receptive listening, you make it safe enough for her to open and connect. This is the same as when you approach yourself with kindness. Inquiring with kindness makes it possible for you to contact your own inner ability to be present and heal.

Realize Non-identification and Nurture Yourself

The "N" of RAIN represents the freedom of Non-identification, which means that you can recognize that what is happening is happening because of conditions you find yourself in. The thoughts, beliefs, feelings, and body sensations are all present to make it happen. But, it's not *who* you are. "Non-identification means that your sense of who you are is not fused with or defined by any limited set of emotions, sensations or stories. When identification with the small self is loosened, we begin to intuit and live from the openness and love that express our natural awareness," says Tara Brach (2018). Once you realize that this present feeling is both a product of conditions and is impermanent, you can truly rest and let it be.

You let go of needing to do something about it and you rest in this natural awareness.

The "N" also reminds you to Nurture yourself. Continue to offer yourself understanding and kindness for having the experience you are having.

Now it's time to practice with the GMATI-3 meditation. As you are turning toward any difficult emotions that have to do with your insomnia, try bringing some RAIN to your experience.

***

When you are through, take some time to journal and reflect on what you noticed. Now, remembering that nonjudgment is at the heart of mindfulness, what did you notice:

- In your body?

- In your mind?

- And in your mood?

Day 5: Stages of Progress

You've been working with the GMATI meditations for eighteen days already, and you may be noticing improvement in your sleep. But it is also still possible that you may be doubting whether mindfulness and self-compassion can make any difference in how you're struggling with anxiety related to insomnia. Today's theme is here to let you know that if you are having that feeling, it may mean you are making progress—as you will see! And, of course, we are not done with offering you help.

Developing a mindfulness and self-compassion practice has three stages (Neff and Germer, 2018):

- Striving.

- Disillusionment.

- Radical acceptance.

We all start with *striving.* You want to sleep better! You want to feel better! That is your intention and that is striving. And meditation practice can in the beginning leave you feeling very relaxed and at peace, which makes you feel better. It may even be helping you sleep a bit better.

But it's a little like the infatuation stage of a romantic relationship. Like any relationship, *disillusionment* can quickly follow when we realize that "it doesn't always *work* to get me feeling relaxed and to sleep!" This is when you realize that you may have been using meditation as a "trick" to get you to sleep because it may have happened once or twice. You start trying to manipulate your moment-to-moment experience to create a specific outcome, and this ultimately only engenders *resistance.* Meditation has become a *technique,* and all techniques are destined to fail. When you use mindfulness and self-compassion to manipulate your mental state, the practice has been hijacked. And then, when that state is not achieved, you feel disillusioned. It's not a problem of mindfulness or self-compassion itself, but more a problem of intention.

There is a saying in mindful self-compassion classes: "We don't give ourselves compassion to transcend suffering, but because we *are* suffering." This saying can be really helpful because it shows you where you might be striving and trying to "make" something happen other than what is happening in the moment.

Once you realize that you may have been caught in this cycle, you can start to experience radical *acceptance.* This is where compassion is so needed. But you are no longer throwing compassion at yourself to make insomnia go away. Rather, you are letting your heart melt into compassion when it encounters the pain and difficulty that is created by insomnia. You let go of the struggle and you just bring acceptance and kindness to yourself. The paradox might be that that's when your mind and body can actually rest better, because there is no longer a constant battle with insomnia going on inside.

So now, reflect on where you might be finding yourself. Wherever you are at in the experience of using mindfulness and self-compassion to support you in dealing with insomnia, know that you are in a process. Each stage is important and can teach you something. But realize that these stages are not at all going to flow in a straight line. You will likely cycle through them again and again at different times.

Now it's time to practice with the GMATI-3 meditation.

***

When you are finished, take another moment to reflect on what your experience was. Now, remembering that nonjudgment is at the heart of mindfulness, what did you notice:

- In your body?

- In your mind?

- And in your mood?

Day 6: Unplugging from FOMO

Do you ever feel like you are being bombarded every day with more and more demands on your attention? You may even still be struggling with how to fit in the meditations in this book, let alone all the other things you have to do in your work and home life. And now add on top of all that the invitation to "let go!" There's so much to "let go" of! Sound familiar?

First of all, it is really amazing that we can experience our lives as so full that we can't find ten or twenty minutes to spend with ourselves to cultivate mindfulness. Being a human being in the modern developed world can be extremely busy! Home demands, work demands, family responsibilities, and on and on. Too often we juggle it all with the pace of a frenetic bee and we rely on technology to help us. But, in addition to the complicated ways we keep ourselves very busy and with all our fancy gadgets that are designed to supposedly increase communication and bring more convenience to our lives, we have inadvertently sworn fealty to small electronic masters that rule our lives and time. They beep, ding, and constantly beckon for attention. We experience extreme FOMO (Fear Of Missing Out) and have developed all sorts of compulsions around needing to check our devices constantly. In Chinese medicine, there is a teaching that says: "Where attention goes, energy follows." This means that every time we shift our attention to the myriad messages and to-do's that our devices demand, we are sending energy out. No wonder we're exhausted all the time!

We live in a time when we are never apart from devices that are demanding our attention. Notifications call out to us in a steady stream, announcing the news, a new message, something nifty to buy, and how the weather is changing. We have no lack of ways to be in constant connectivity to the entire world around us. All these alerts demand that we respond in some way, bringing knowledge, yes, but along with it the stress to *do* something. So while we are gaining increasing opportunity to relate to everything outside ourselves, we are losing the ability to be in relationship to our own body, mind, and heart. There is a passage in the New Testament that says "You gain the whole world, yet lose and forfeit your very self." Is that what is happening to us? With mindfulness, we can become truly intimate with all things, including the landscape of our own hearts and minds.

But FOMO, and the chronic impulse to be "doing something" or to feel like something is wrong with us or missing from our lives, didn't just start with advancements in smartphone technology. We have been conditioned to evaluate our worth by how much we get done, or how productive we are. And so this nagging drive to "do something" pokes at us around the clock and seems in direct opposition to "letting go."

Even sleep can feel like something we have to "do better." You may have read all the books on sleep hygiene and tried all the tricks to make sleep happen. And when it doesn't, you feel like you have failed again! And so at this point in reading this book, you may be still thinking: "How the heck am I going to find time to practice meditation when I already feel so maxed out and exhausted?" It, too, can feel like one more thing you *have* to do! That mindset makes you even more stressed out.

The news is full of articles about how to develop a more healthy and balanced relationship with technology. The full breadth of that subject is beyond the scope of this book, but in the spirit of letting go, we do need to look at how the addiction to technology has an impact on sleep, and a few things we can do differently, so we can develop a more conscientious relationship to the onslaught of stimuli that exists in modern life and learn to "unplug" during the day and then wind down into rest at the end of our day. Here are some ways you can do just that!

1. Throughout the day, try mindfully pausing before you answer your phone or respond to a notification. Notice whether there is any tension in your mind or body and then take a deep breath before you move on to interacting with your phone.

2. In the moments when you feel the tug to engage in social media, pause and see what is happening inside you—in your mind, body, and mood. If there is boredom or restlessness, see if you can be with that for a few breaths before just reflexively diving into filling your attention with whatever the social media outlet supplies.

3. Have a cutoff time for work emails. It's true that you get a little blip of adrenaline every time you get a request that requires a response. Defending a boundary about how late you'll work can sometimes feel like a big ask, but it will benefit your work, and your sleep overall.

4. Start winding down the brain and body by dimming the lights an hour before bedtime. Engage in relaxing activities outside the bedroom that pass the time quietly.

5. Use the time before bed to do some of the stretches you practiced in Weeks 2 and 3. Create a quiet space and let yourself be guided by the recording. Or make up your own sequence of relaxing stretches while listening to some gentle music.

6. Create a bedtime ritual. It might be mindfully taking a bath, brushing your teeth, and reading for half an hour by a gentle light. Establishing a set routine and sticking to it means you're less likely to be exposed to unpredictable thoughts right before you hit the hay. Excluding your phone from that ritual isn't a bad idea either.

7. Avoid looking at anything with a screen. Stow away your tablet, phone, computer, and TV for the night—the light can keep you awake and alert. Sleep with your phone in another room. It sounds obvious, but getting hold of an old-fashioned alarm clock and leaving your cellphone someplace else when you go to bed might give you a little more space. At the very least, you won't be tempted to reach for your phone when you can't sleep. If you are planning on using you phone to listen to a meditation, make sure it is in airplane mode so that you won't be disturbed.

8. Ten minutes before bedtime, begin any of the mindfulness practices you have learned throughout this book to continue winding down.

And one of the most helpful things you can do is to cultivate mindfulness and the ability to be in a wise and kind relationship to yourself. Throughout the day, try writing down any times you notice the pull to engage with technology or the impulse to be "accomplishing" something, in order to more fully understand how this shows up for you. Have some compassion for yourself for how conditioned this tug is, and use it as an opportunity to develop a more mindful or skillful way to relate to the technology in your life.

So, now it's time to use the GMATI-3 meditation.

***

When you have finished, take some time to be with yourself and note what you experienced. Now, remembering that nonjudgment is at the heart of mindfulness, what did you notice:

- In your body?

- In your mind?

- And in your mood?

Day 7: Meditation as an Act of Love

Dear reader, you've been doing a lot this week. It's day 7, and we want you to have time to integrate all this learning—all these ways that you have been turning toward feeling and experiencing the thoughts and emotions and other stimuli related to your insomnia. This takes tremendous valor.

So today, the main guidance we have is for you to spend your time in meditation with wholehearted warmth and affection toward yourself. See your meditation as an act of love. As a time to be with yourself and care for all of the facets of your mind and heart. A time to skillfully utilize the various supports you've encountered these past few weeks as you attend to the unfolding of each and every moment.

Allow yourself to really be held by whatever you are resting on, and by your own kind attention. Allow yourself to experience the reserves of courage you have that enable you to be with all of your changing thoughts and emotions and body sensations. Experience them, and then let them go. Try to be like a body of water, where, regardless of the intensity of waves on the surface, at the bottom, there are only gentle undulations of current or even reservoirs of stillness. You could see your own thoughts and feelings like the waves. They arise because of conditions and weather, and then they go. But beneath it all, there is a stillness and a peace that you can count on and experience.

Now, it's time to again practice with the GMATI-3 meditation. See if you can invite a feeling of internal spaciousness and receptivity as you work with whatever arises for you.

***

When you have finished, take some time to be with yourself and note what you experienced. Now, remembering that nonjudgment is at the heart of mindfulness, what did you notice:

- In your body?

- In your mind?

- And in your mood?

Now you are ready to move on to the final week of this GMATI sequence.

CHAPTER 7

GMATI—Week 4

In Week 1, we had you spend time experiencing mindful awareness, and in Week 2, you took up practices that were about helping you to "accept" what is happening with your insomnia. Then last week, in Week 3 of the GMATI program, you got a taste of "letting go." And now here we are in the Week 4.

It's not easy to change habits, and so we want to take a minute to allow you to really recognize all that you have done so far to make time for meditation and all the practices in this book. That's a lot! If you have been practicing, you are building momentum. And the amazing thing is that, once you set the mindfulness ball in motion, and keep tending to it, it's impossible for it not to have some effects. Any time you change the conditions in your mind and heart, you have change. This doesn't mean that you can always see these changes immediately. You may be sleeping better, but on the other hand, you may not, yet. That is okay. What you are doing with bringing mindfulness into your day will have an effect at night. You know that's true in reverse—that what happens at night affects your day.

So think about it as planting seeds. Inside a live seed is all the potential for it to transform into whatever plant it was meant to become. All it needs is for the soil to be watered, nurtured, and allowed to get some sunshine. The seed operates under natural laws. So does mindfulness. In time, you will see it as being able to have a little more perspective on things, and you will find yourself being a little less reactive to what is happening. You may also notice yourself relating to yourself with more friendliness and compassion. And with all of this, you may find that those "right box" factors we wrote about back in chapter 3 are becoming less of a problem, and that you are resting more easily.

Another metaphor for how mindfulness works is the power of water. It will flow and endlessly continue its journey to the sea. If you've ever visited the Grand Canyon, or other canyons, you can see the incredible power of water to transform the landscape. And so, you have been tending to the garden of your mind and heart with your mindfulness practice. You have been allowing the water of mindfulness to flow. We're really proud of you and hope you'll keep it up!

Week 4

You have been encouraged for the last three weeks to focus on doing mindfulness practice in the daytime and letting that mindfulness indirectly improve your sleep. And that is still vitally important. The theme for this week is to help you to continue developing *confidence* in your ability to sleep. So in addition to the fourth and final GMATI formal meditation, which you should continue to practice during the day, we will be giving you some exercises you can do without formal practice and without listening to a guided recording. The fourth GMATI meditation is one that helps to tie together everything you have done so far. Simply put, practicing mindfulness is remembering to recognize the present moment just as it is. You recognize the present moment as just as it is because the conditions were there for whatever *is* happening to *be* happening. There's no need to add anything to what's already there or to try to make it be any other way. That only adds stress, and stress doesn't help you experience rest.

But another major theme for this week is broadening how you can work toward developing more confidence in your ability to sleep! Sleep is a natural process, and your work with mindfulness allows you to create the conditions for it to happen naturally. You are now ready to start skillfully (but carefully) learning how to use mindfulness at nighttime when you can't sleep, in order to help your mindfulness practice calm your mind, heart, and body to assist your sleep.

It's important to know what you can use to support yourself in the middle of the night if you find yourself awake. By now you know that you're not doing these things to *make* yourself fall asleep. They are simply there to remind your mind and heart to relax and be at ease with whatever *is* happening. There is no "trick" in mindfulness. You practice mindfulness so that you can assist yourself in having more compassion and ease with yourself, which may then help you accept being awake or help with falling sleep.

When you bring mindfulness into your bed on nights when you can't sleep, you are calling on the attitudes that you have learned in these weeks of practicing the GMATI meditations during the day: acknowledging, accepting, and letting go. And when you do this, you are learning a new way of being in bed when sleep eludes you. You are not "struggling" with insomnia, you are simply noting whatever conditions are present and letting them be as they are. The more you do this, the more confidence you will gain in being able to bring ease and rest to your mind and body. If in doing so you fall asleep, fine. If not, fine. A night spent in meditation is much better for the mind and body than a night spent fighting insomnia.

So this week, we'll highlight reminders of what you can use to remember to bring compassionate awareness to yourself at night, and additional suggestions that you might find helpful to support yourself during the night when sleep is not coming easily. It's not necessary to use a guided recording for these. Rather, we strongly recommend that you guide yourself, in order to flex that muscle of mindfully befriending yourself and to know your own ability to bring support to your mind and body.

We still want you to meditate during waking hours using a GMATI meditation. Here is the meditation for Week 4. As before, it's helpful to read it through now. As you do so, pause every now and again and feel what kind of impact the words are having right then and there. When you're through reading it, you'll find a recorded version on the New Harbinger website (http://www.newharbinger.com/42587), which you can use to guide your meditation. Enjoy the practice!

GMATI-4 MEDITATION

As you begin this meditation, take a moment to establish yourself as best you can in a posture that embodies dignity, whether you are sitting on a chair, on the floor, or lying down. Allow the eyes to be either open with the gaze stable and unfocused in front of you or gently closed. Establish a gentle and firm intention to be as present as possible—to have this time for yourself. Being as in touch as possible with the present moment, just as it is and however it is for you, using these words merely as guidance in the process. What is important is your experience. You can tune out or drop underneath the spoken guidance at any time, in order to focus on your own experience, both during the speaking and during the stretches of silence.

At this time, allow the awareness to notice the body as a whole. Bring into the center stage of your awareness sensations of touch—all of the places in which your body makes contact with the chair or cushion, contact made by the feet, by the buttocks, by the legs—as you sit in a posture that exemplifies presence and dignity.

Let these sensations of contact give you the message that in this moment, the body is held and supported, so you can really settle in, be at ease, and allow yourself to experience that support.

You may also notice the feelings at the periphery of the body—feeling into the space where the body ends and where the space around you begins. Feeling that the body is in fact in a very dynamic relationship to space, because it is breathing. Breath comes in and the body expands, breath goes out and the body recedes and settles once again, continually flowing with the in and out, with expansion and release.

Let the sensations of breath emerge into the foreground of your attention. Not shutting out other experiences around you, but simply allowing the breath to be center stage, aware of the movement of the breath, as it comes into the body, and as it *leaves* the body. Now, focus on some region in the body where the breath sensations are most vivid for you right now. Perhaps noticing the sensations of the breath in the belly or chest, feeling the abdomen *rising* as the breath moves into the body, and *falling* as it moves out of the body. Or at the nostrils, where you're actually feeling the passage of the air as it comes in and out. Or a larger sense of the entirety of the breath, from the nostrils down to the belly, or any other place in the body where the sensations of breath are vivid for you. And without forcing or striving, as best you can, just ride on the waves of your own breathing, moment by moment, as a leaf might ride on the surface of a stream.

If you notice that the breath is no longer in the foreground of your attention, and has perhaps been replaced with thoughts of planning, fantasy, or memory, simply and intentionally escort your focus, your attention, back to the breathing. Picking up wherever it happens to be—on an in-breath or on an out-breath—just observing, moving up close to your breathing, fully present with the duration of this *in-breath,* and with the duration of this *out-breath,* from moment to moment.

Now, letting the sensations of the breath recede into the background of your awareness, begin noticing sensations from elsewhere within your body. Sensations of temperature, sensations of the body sitting, or whatever other sensations present themselves—sensations arising, perhaps lingering or changing in intensity, or passing away. Being aware of your body as a whole and of whatever sensations or feelings are coming up in any moment.

Being here with whatever does come up, without judging it, without reacting to it, just *being fully here,* fully aware. Maybe saying to yourself "*Oh, it's like this now."* Totally present with whatever feelings present themselves, and with a sense of your body as a *complete, dignified whole.*

Whenever you notice that the mind may have wandered off, just bring it back to your breathing, and to a sense of the body as you sit here. Not going anywhere, not doing anything, simply being, simply sitting, from moment to moment, being fully present with yourself just as you are in *this* moment.

Now, as you sit here, once again, allow the field of your awareness to expand. This time, let the attention move toward hearing, toward sounds you may be aware of in the environment, or from within your own body. Imagine that you have the ears of a doe, large, receptive, and open. Bring into the foreground of your attention the sensations of hearing, of receiving sound in the ears. Not going out searching for things to hear, but simply being receptive to whatever it is that enters your awareness as sound. *Full* awareness of hearing from *one* moment to the next.

When you do hear a sound of whatever kind, see if you can let go of the tendency to judge, identify, or evaluate it. Let go of deciding whether you like it or dislike it. Simply reside in the moment-to-moment experience of being with hearing, with sounds. Sitting in stillness, aware of sound, and aware of the space between sounds. Sounds arising and passing into silence, *moment by moment.*

Again, if the mind becomes caught up in thinking, or other body sensations, if it moves away from sound, just recognize that this has happened and bring it back to your breathing or to your ears, to anchor yourself. Bring your attention back to right now, and to whatever you're hearing as you sit here.

Now, as you sit here, let your awareness of hearing move into the background and once again allow the field of your awareness to expand. This time we will expand the awareness to include *thinking* and *feeling*. To include thoughts and feelings as they move through the mind rather than considering them as distractions in your attention. Being open to the experience of thinking and feeling.

Let your breathing, your sense of the body and of sounds, be in the background, and allow the thinking and feeling processes *themselves* to come into the foreground of your awareness. As if your thoughts and feelings were the clouds drifting by in the blue sky. Observe each thought, each feeling as it *comes* up from the mind, aware of each as it moves *across* the field of awareness, arising, perhaps moving through the awareness quickly, perhaps lingering then passing away. Just as if they were clouds of different sizes, different shapes, different thicknesses, different masses, moving across the sky, each thought, each emotion an observable event, coming, drifting by, going.

Any time you find yourself caught by a thought, caught in the content of a thought, or caught in a stream of thoughts, or caught in a story—as soon as you realize this has happened, note that that's what has occurred, and then come back to just observing, using the breathing and a sense of your body to anchor yourself, to stabilize yourself in the present before opening back up to observing thoughts.

You could even try counting the thoughts. As you become aware of a thought arising, just lightly, as if you were touching a bubble with a feather, giving the thought a number. One ... two ... and so on, gently whispering the number to yourself when you notice the presence of a thought.

Of course, thoughts can take any form, they can have any content. They can be neutral or they can be highly charged. And in particular, if thoughts or emotions come up about sleep, just be aware that that's what's here. Perhaps it's fear or anxiety or concerns about what tomorrow might be like. You might say to yourself, *"Oh, it's like this now."* You're just being aware of *the thought or emotion* as a momentary occurrence. Becoming aware of it *coming* and *going.* The same for worries or preoccupations of one kind or another, or pressures in the mind, the thought of deadlines or obligations, even thoughts like *"I'm a bad meditator."* And again, regardless of the *charge* that the thought has for you, just observe it as a discrete mental event, and just let it be here, without pursuing it or rejecting it. And noticing, of course, that from moment to moment, new thoughts will come *and go.*

Now, for the remaining time, let go of all deliberate objects of attention, all of your breathing, your body, your hearing, your thinking, your feeling. Not deciding ahead of time to focus on any one thing. Simply allow yourself to sit here, fully present, fully *aware* in each moment, aware of whatever is presenting itself in this moment. If thoughts come, observe those thoughts. If sounds come, observe those sounds. If pain is present, observe the pain. If the breath is predominant, then be with the breath, looking for nothing. Being sensitive and present with it *all,* just as it is, just as it *unfolds.* Perhaps periodically noting to yourself, as a way of connecting with presence, "*Oh, it's like this now.*"

Experience the *ground of being,* experience the ground of awareness, out of which *all* perceptions arise. Being *right* here with it. Complete as you are. Human. Whole.

And now, gather in the focus of your awareness once again and bring your attention back to the breath, the anchor of the breath, becoming aware of the breath as it moves *into* the body, and as it moves *out* of the body. Riding the *flow* of the breath with your attention. Being fully present with each in-breath, and with each out-breath. Breathing. Nothing you need to do, only to be fully present with each breath, moving *into* the body, moving *out* of the body.

As the meditation comes to a close, recognize that you have spent this time intentionally nourishing yourself by dwelling in this state of nondoing. This state of *being,* this state of *intentionally* making time for you to be who you are, just as you are, in the unfolding moments of your life, moment by moment by moment.

Day 1: Gladdening the Mind and Soothing Touch

Over these last three weeks, you have been learning practices that are all aimed at helping you experience less stress and reactivity in your life, especially in relation to your sleep. But thoughts, perceptions, and attitudes about insomnia are just one of the ways we humans can get ourselves all tangled up. You may already be noticing that there are many thoughts that can cause the body, emotions, and mind to tense up. As the clock ticks throughout the day and night, all those tensions accumulate, and pretty soon, you're walking around with a full coat of stress and tension-related "body armor." When that is the case, you swing between losing access to the sensitivity of the heart and the wisdom it contains to feeling totally vulnerable and like a ticking time bomb. It's easy then to pingpong back and forth between the two extremes. Add thoughts of helplessness and self-criticism to that mix, and the next thing you know, you are bound up in suffering and definitely not sleeping well.

So, as we go along over these weeks, start to really pay attention to what kinds of thoughts cause stress and tension. You may see that there are certain ones that are not really helpful, and others that are. With a mindfulness practice, you start to learn about what's happening inside yourself—what are the causes of stress that you can influence, and what are the causes for release? Once you see that a thought or reaction that is present is stressful, you can ask yourself, "Do I really need to be holding on to these thoughts right now?" Maybe they were useful at some point, but when they play over and over in a loop, they just cause suffering. And by now, because of what you have practiced, you've begun to see that thoughts are discreet events that you can notice and relate to, and even let go of. The question remains, "What then are the kinds of thoughts that help the mind and body be at ease?" And that's what you're going to explore in part today.

Here's an experiment:

Start by noticing how you feel right now—in your body, mind, and mood. No need to judge anything; just check out what is present for you right now.

Now make a list, either mentally or by writing it down, of at least twenty things you appreciate in your life. There's no need to make it grand or complicated. Things like "popcorn," or "my dog," or "sunshine on my back" will do.

After you have made your list, read it over again and take time to let the feelings of appreciation and gladness seep into your heart. Now, tune back in to your body, mind, and mood. How do you feel now? Do you see how you can intentionally gladden your heart by simply shifting your attention for a little bit to thoughts that are nourishing?

Sometimes your body can respond to nourishing care more quickly than your mind. So another way to increase a sense of relaxation and openness to yourself is through the power of touch. Think about what you yourself do when you are with someone you care about or who is struggling in some way. Or what you like to receive when you are suffering and someone connects with you. Often, there is a strong impulse to reach out, hold a hand, or give a soothing hug. In fact, soothing touch is one of the two universal triggers of compassion (the other is gentle vocalizations) (Steller and Keltner, 2014). When you give yourself physical gestures of self-compassion, you can generate a sense of safety and comfort within yourself. This is possible because, as mammals, we are hardwired to feel soothed and safe when we receive these compassion triggers. When the mammalian care-giving system is activated through compassionate interaction, oxytocin and endogenous opiates are released in the body, and this can counteract the stress that is created when the threat-defense system gets turned on.

You tried this back in Week 2 of the GMATI program when we introduced you to the "self-compassion break." For many people, having a hand or both hands resting on the heart feels soothing, but for others, it might not. See if you can let yourself experience the comfort that you can give to your own body and heart—try out a few of the gestures below and see if any resonate with you.

- Take a moment to settle into your seat and take a few deep breaths. Allow your eyes to close and then try each of these gestures. Really take your time to breathe with the gesture and feel whatever you are feeling.

- Gently place a hand against your cheek.

- Now, try cradling your face in both of your hands.

- Gently stroke down your arm. Try doing the down stroke along with your out-breath.

- Cross your arms across your body and give a gentle squeeze.

- Make a gentle fist with one hand and place it over your heart, and then cup your other hand over it.

- Gently stroke your chest by going back and forth or making little circles around your heart.

- Place one hand over your belly and one over your heart.

- Place both hands over your belly.

- Let both hands rest in your lap and cradle one hand in the other.

These gestures can be a really helpful to use at night when you are having trouble sleeping. By bringing in a gesture of compassion, you are reminding yourself to bring a kind and affectionate awareness to yourself with whatever is happening. Try doing this during any of the GMATI meditations or any meditations that you try using at night in bed.

Now it's time to practice the GMATI-4 meditation. See how it feels to begin with some appreciation and a gesture of compassion.

***

When you have finished the practice, write down some notes in your journal. Remembering that nonjudgment is at the heart of mindfulness, what did you notice:

- In your body?

- In your mind?

- And in your mood?

Day 2: Loving-Kindness Meditation

As we've begun to explore in the last few days, whatever your mind is chewing on will have an impact on your mood, your outlook, and how your body feels. Today's practice, called loving-kindness meditation, is a way of training the mind to be more loving and compassionate. What you think about is what you think about. The more you consciously develop a compassionate mind state through this meditation, the more compassion becomes a personal trait that can be extremely beneficial in meeting yourself during the suffering that can come from insomnia, as well as from any other difficulties you may be experiencing. Like all practices, it is somewhat "dose" dependent; that is, the more you do, the more easily accessible it is and the more reliable the effects. In this practice, as in the self-compassion break you practiced in Week 2, you are accessing the power of language and using phrases as the primary focus of attention. If you ever doubt the power of words, just consider:

Have you ever broken a bone?

Has it healed?

Have you ever been hurt by the words of another?

Are you still suffering from harsh words that were said to you years ago?

You may want to consider this saying: "Be careful what you say to yourself, because you are listening!"

So in this practice, you are harnessing the power of (1) language, (2) imagery, (3) concentration, (4) connection, and (5) caring. The concentration aspect of this meditation leads to calmness and relaxation, but loving-kindness meditation also calms by directly offering comfort and soothing.

You are also building a good and positive internal conversation with yourself, which can lead to a better mood state. Your intentions drive your internal conversation. So if you find yourself awake in the middle of the night and need a good "friend" to be there for you, you can do that for yourself with this practice. It's a whole lot better than lying there berating yourself over and over for not sleeping and imagining that you'll never sleep well again.

You can find a recording of this meditation on the New Harbinger website (http://www.newharbinger.co m/42587); but for now, just read along and get a sense for how it goes.

> Allow yourself to settle into a comfortable position. Perhaps placing a hand over your heart or another location that is soothing, as a reminder to bring not only awareness, but a loving awareness to your experience, and to yourself. Take a few breaths and feel that you are safe, right where you are.

> Now, bring to mind some person from your life who naturally makes you smile. Someone with whom you have an easy, uncomplicated relationship. This could be a grandparent, a child, a beloved teacher or friend, or even your cat or dog—whoever naturally brings a feeling of delight and happiness to your heart and a smile to your face. Just let yourself feel what it is like to be in that being's presence. Create as vivid an image in your mind as possible and just feel what it's like to revel in that good company.

It is natural to have within your heart hopes and wishes for this person to be happy and free from suffering. Every being has these same longings—including this one you are holding in your heart, and you yourself as well. Allow these wishes to take the form of silent expressions, as if you could beam these wishes of good will from your heart to theirs. Repeating softly and gently:

May you be safe.

May you be happy.

May you be healthy.

May you live with ease and peace.

Just continue to repeat these phrases, sending these wishes to your dear one. These phrases address some of our most fundamental and universal needs. We all desire to be safe: safe and protected from harm, safe in our bodies, in our minds, and in our spirits. We all desire to be happy. Not just "got a new car happy," but deeply and fundamentally happy. We all long to be as healthy as we possibly can in our bodies, minds, and spirits. And there is not a being alive who doesn't long for peace and to have a life that is unobstructed by struggles and full of ease. And so that's why you can use these phrases. But you may wish to use your own words to capture your deepest wishes for your loved one. Find some inner whispering that expresses a wish that your loved one's deepest longings be met and satisfied.

When you notice that your mind has wandered (because inevitably it will), simply acknowledge that and return to the words and the image of the loved one you have in mind, savoring any warm feelings that may arise. And remember to take your time.

Now, after some time sending these wishes in the direction of your friend, see what it's like to add yourself to this circle of good will you have created. Try creating an image of yourself right alongside your loved one, visualizing the both of you together. Imagine scooping up a cupful of good will that you've cultivated, and spread it to the both of you. Saying now:

May you and I (we) be safe.

May you and I (we) be happy.

May you and I (we) be healthy.

May you and I (we) live with ease and peace.

Continue repeating these offerings for a little bit and then let the image of your friend move into the background of your circle, as if the friend was standing behind you. You can even thank your friend before moving on, now letting the full focus of your attention rest directly on yourself. Place your hand over your heart and feel the warmth and gentle pressure of making kind contact with yourself. Visualize your whole body in your mind's eye, noticing any stress or uneasiness that may be lingering within you, and offering yourself the phrases:

May I be safe.

May I be happy.

May I be healthy.

May I live with ease and peace.

Spend some time with yourself in this way, allowing these phrases to be scooped up from the fount of loving-kindness that you have been cultivating and pouring them into your own heart.

Finally, take a few breaths and rest quietly in your own body, accepting whatever your experience is, exactly as it is.

This can be an extremely powerful practice to use both formally, when listening to the recording, and informally when doing this on your own. When loving-kindness is present in the mind and heart, you are more at ease. This practice should be effortless. So if you find yourself struggling to feel something profound or to send just the "right" message, simply let go. The language is here to help you connect with your intrinsic capacity to experience good will, but it is not something to get too hung up about. If the words that we've offered don't resonate with you, no worries. It may even be enough to just experience the tenderness of the heart when you call to mind someone you care about. The smile that may come to your mouth and the possible feelings of warmth, openness, and ease in your chest reflect the arising of lovingkindness. You can just mentally hang out there.

Some people even like to imagine the feelings, great or subtle, of loving-kindness as if they are a light beam that they mentally shine in the direction of others. This can be a really helpful way to either start or end any of the meditations you are already doing. It can also be used when you're driving and want to send good will to the other drivers around you. Or maybe try sending some loving-kindness to your fellow shoppers when you're in a long line at the grocery store or at the bank. You can also send loving-kindness to yourself and others as you lie in your bed. No need to make it a big formal thing. You can just incline your mind toward this inner friendliness and give loving-kindness to yourself and anyone else you choose.

Feel free to listen to the recording as an additional formal practice to your daily GMATI meditation. But once you get the hang of it, just try ending your GMATI meditation with a few minutes of loving-kindness.

And now it's time to practice the GMATI-4 meditation, using the recording at the New Harbinger website (h ttp://www.newharbinger.com/42587).

***

When you are finished, try to enjoy time reflecting on what you noticed during and after the meditation. Remembering that nonjudgment is at the heart of mindfulness, what are you noticing:

- In your body?

- In your mind?

- And in your mood?

Day 3: Mindful Self-Guidance at Night

Here we are in the middle of the last week of this four-week series! You have learned a lot and have developed many skills to cultivate mindfulness and get better rest. The theme this week is to enhance your confidence in your ability to sleep, which has been developing because of your work with mindfulness. An additional theme that you may have noticed is that even if you are not sleeping as easily or as often as you like, you may be experiencing more acceptance and less struggle during those nights. That in itself is an incredible benefit. The less the struggle, the more conditioned a peaceful repose will be, and that *will* lead to better sleep.

In this book, you have been receiving so many practices and instructions that at times, you may feel bombarded by more meditations to "do." So today, we're just going to have a little chat and remember some things. All the meditation practices that we've offered are aimed at the cultivation of mindfulness and compassion. In themselves, they are just tools. You already have the capacity inside yourself for both mindful attention and compassion. Yes, practicing the tools helps develop these qualities, but remember that the point of meditating is not to just be a good meditator. It's really important that you feel your own confidence in your ability to be mindful and at ease with the changing nature of life.

Over these last few weeks, you have been encouraged to practice the meditations during the day rather than using them as a technique for falling asleep. So we believe you understand the importance of that distinction. Today and for the next few days, we'll be turning our attention to ways that you can be with yourself during the middle of the night when you find yourself awake. When this happens, it can be a good time to bring mindfulness and compassion into your consciousness. Be sure to remember that you are not doing this to make yourself fall asleep. It's possible you will fall asleep, but if you don't, that's okay! Lying awake in a state of peaceful, gentle mindfulness is good too.

There are times when your innate mindfulness, or ability to focus on the present moment with kindness, is obscured. Like rocks blocking a pathway. These "rocks" or obscurations can take many forms. Unfortunately, fatigue and having a mind that is either foggy or anxious can make present-moment awareness challenging. And these states may be the ones you encounter in the middle of the night when you can't sleep.

Since you've been doing lots of meditation practice during the day over these past few weeks, your "path" of mindfulness is getting well grooved in and clear. But let's look at some additional ways you can remember to call up this nonjudgmental awareness when you encounter some "rocks" along the path at night.

The first might be to develop a clear association with something in your bed—such as your pillow or a blanket—that helps you return to the present moment and connect with the feeling of your body and your breath. You can use this object as a cue to help your mind remember to return to yourself with a kind and gentle attention. It's the "remembering" that is often the hardest thing about developing mindfulness, and so whatever you can do to just start making it an automatic habit will help.

Also, pay attention to the language that resonates with you as you listen to the guided practices. See what phrases and instructions help you settle into yourself and into presence. Then, guide yourself, as best you can, through a meditation. You are becoming your own teacher. You are becoming your own inner ally and support. Continue to let the momentum of mindfulness carve out its channels of peace in your mind, heart, and body.

Practice during the day to continually remind yourself of these ways of being with the breath and body to create the conditions for ease. If, throughout the entire time, you are guiding yourself you remain awake, no worries. Just take the time to be mindful of being calm and quiet in your bed, and seek solace in the fact that you are conserving energy for the day ahead.

Now it's time again to practice the GMATI-4 meditation.

***

When you have finished, take some time to be with yourself and note what you experienced. Now, remembering that nonjudgment is at the heart of mindfulness, what did you notice:

- In your body?

- In your mind?

- And in your mood?

Day 4: Nighttime Imagery for the Monkey Mind

One of the biggest challenges people report with insomnia is that their mind just won't "shut off" when they want to go to sleep or return to sleep. Even if you are exhausted at the end of the day and can barely keep your eyes open to brush your teeth, the minute your head hits the pillow, it's as if a switch gets turned on and your mind is like a monkey, frantically swinging from thought to thought or to the same thing over and over again. You've been practicing for almost four weeks now on how to work with "monkey mind" through all of the GMATI meditations and other practices. All the meditations you have done up to this point can help the tension that can get created from monkey mind, and you've been learning what you can do with your attention when you experience this. If you've been practicing daily, you are likely very familiar with the different modes of the mind and have developed some skill both in redirecting your attention and in accepting that this happens.

Today, we'll look at some additional imagery you can work with to help you during the day and then use at night if you find that your mind is really active. It's not that different from what you've already learned, but the specific imagery can be useful for some people when they struggle to relate to thoughts as "events." So just give it a try and see if it helps.

Earlier, you were introduced to an imagery exercise that included some flowing water. That can be a really helpful metaphor for the "stream of thoughts" that flow through the mind.

Imagine now that you are sitting on the edge or bank of a slowly moving stream. On the surface of the stream leaves are floating by.

Let this image form in your mind's eye. Let it really come into form. Hanging out in your imagination, try looking around. What do you see? Is the stream moving from the left or the right? Is the sun shining or is the moon out? Is the water smooth or wavy? Now, during these next few moments, take every thought that shows up in your mind and place it on a leaf in the stream, and let it float on by. Do this regardless of the content of the thought, whether positive or negative, comfortable or uncomfortable. Even if the most wonderful thoughts begin to show up, gently place them on a leaf and let them float away with the stream.

Every now and again, a thought may try to hook you, and you may lose contact with the imagery. This is not a problem. It may even happen over and over again. No big deal. As soon as you realize that this has happened, gently note it and just return to the practice of placing your thoughts on the leaves traveling in the current of the stream.

You may even notice a gap or pause in the thoughts, and then you can simply just observe the stream floating by. Sooner or later, another thought will show up.

Let the stream float on by at its own pace. Don't try to rush it. You are not trying to flush the leaves away, but just letting them pass on by at their own pace. If you notice a thought or leaf getting stuck, let it linger. Don't force it to float away. It will gently get unstuck and move on on its own.

It may happen that an uncomfortable feeling arises, like boredom or restlessness. Just notice the feeling, and try saying to yourself, "Here is a feeling of boredom" or "Here is a feeling of restlessness." And then, gently place those words or thoughts on a leaf too, and let them float on down the stream as well.

See if this way of addressing thoughts helps you develop a healthy distance from them and assists you in just being able to observe them. This can be extremely helpful when you are experiencing a rascally nocturnal monkey mind and it's keeping you up. Also, feel free to use this as you now go ahead and practice with the GMATI-4 meditation.

***

When you're through, take note of what you experienced. Remembering that nonjudgment is at the heart of mindfulness, what did you notice:

- In your body?

- In your mind?

- And in your mood?

Day 5: Affectionate Awareness

Many people find that doing a body scan (where you focus your attention on each part of the body in succession, as was emphasized in the GMATI Week 2 meditation) when you are having difficulty going or returning to sleep is another great way to bring a peaceful and kind attention to yourself that can be conducive to rest. But remember that you're doing this not to make sleep magically happen, but more to have a seamlessness to your cultivation of mindfulness—going from day to night.

What follows are some additional attitudes and mental supports you can bring into your experience when you practice the body scan, or any of the other practices where you are paying attention to sensations in the body. You can even do this practice in your bed, in whatever position you find comfortable. Start by taking three slow, relaxing breaths in which you elongate your inhale and exhale. Then, bring to mind these four additional elements of warmth and good will with which you can permeate your awareness when the focus of your meditation is on your body. They will help you along the way.

Gratitude

The body is an incredibly symphony of inner workings. Most of them operate outside of our conscious control—thank goodness! Imagine if you had to remember to breathe! So try bringing in some gratitude for the selfless work of each body part, reflecting for a moment on the myriad ways each part of the body works hard to support and enable you to function in your life. In areas where there is an absence of tensions, you might extend some gratitude for discomfort you *don't* have.

Inner Smile

This can be felt as a loving attitude or inclination toward the body. Incline your awareness toward your body in the same way that you might incline toward a young child, or a dear friend, or even a beloved pet. As you move your attention throughout the body, try inwardly smiling toward it as a gesture of recognition or appreciation.

Loving-Kindness

Here, you are offering compassionate language toward your body and yourself. If you have judgments or unpleasant associations with a particular body part, or if you experience physical discomfort, you may wish to place a hand on that part of your body as a gesture of kindness, perhaps imagining warmth and kindness flowing through your hand into your body. If any parts of your body are too difficult to stay with, gently move the attention to another body part for the time being. Just allowing this practice to be as gentle and peaceful as possible.

When you encounter some discomfort, you can imagine releasing any tension and allowing that area to soften, as if it were wrapped in a warm towel. Maybe even addressing the sensations with kind words, such as: "Oh, there's some discomfort here. That's okay for now. May you (sore area of the body) be at ease. May you be well."

Soothing Touch

Just as we practiced earlier in the week, try placing one or both hands over your heart (or any other soothing place) and doing this as a reminder to bring affectionate awareness to yourself throughout the entire practice. Feel the warmth and gentle touch of your hands. When you have paid loving attention to each individual body part, offer to yourself your soothing gesture once again and give your entire body a shower of care and affection.

As you try guiding yourself through a brief body scan at night when you lay down, you just might find that it will give you something productive to do with your mind instead of growing frustrated if you're not sleeping. Think of this like a soothing blanket that you can wrap yourself up in to help you be with yourself, and to be with whatever is happening.

Hopefully, this will give you a little taste of how you can bring an affectionate awareness into your body when you are lying down in your bed. But for now, while you are out of bed, practice with the GMATI-4 meditation and try to call up some of the attitudes we explored today.

***

When you are finished, take note of what you experienced. Remembering that nonjudgment is at the heart of mindfulness, what did you notice:

- In your body?

- In your mind?

- And in your mood?

Day 6: Feeling Safe

We need to believe in our own safety in order to rest. But when the mind is distracted with all that's not going well, we can easily forget what is working. This is why so many of the meditations and teachings we've offered over these weeks have been in the service of helping you feel safe and at ease.

Intentionally turning your mind toward something and shining the light of your attention on a specific thing or attitude can shape how you experience your life in that moment. Throughout the day, you can intentionally look for ways to acknowledge the relative safety of the present moment—whatever is holding you, such as gravity or the air you breathe. Remind yourself that there are "no saber-toothed tigers here right now." Even if the mind is remembering past moments where there was a lack of safety or where there were concerns or predictions about a future where you might not feel safe and at ease, recognize that at this moment, those are just conditioned thoughts. They usually lack substance in the present moment. Even the ability to be mindfully aware of those thoughts is a protective force. So take a few moments to start naming anything you can think of that is, at this moment, providing for your safety and survival. These could be oxygen to breathe, clothing to keep you warm, the stability of the earth beneath you, the work that you have that helps provide for you, food that you eat, and so on. All these often completely unrecognized conditions are there all the time to meet your needs.

Now, see how you feel after spending a few moments inclining the mind toward these beneficial things. There may be more ease, and even a taste of the feeling of safety when appreciation is present.

Try bringing these attitudes with you today as you now practice the GMATI-4 meditation.

***

When you are finished, take note of what you experienced. Remembering that nonjudgment is at the heart of mindfulness, what did you notice:

- In your body?

- In your mind?

- And in your mood?

Day 7: Imagery for Serene Sleep

Now we turn to a more elaborate method for giving your mind something to use to quiet the bombardment of thoughts it may be experiencing that are keeping you awake. This method, too, can support the GMATI meditations you have been using to indirectly improve your sleep. It relies on the fact that when you focus on a pleasant scene that includes several elements and activities, it fills up your conscious mind, making it harder for other thoughts and emotions to get into your mind to keep you awake. The more you can incorporate all your senses into the scene, the better it will do this. However, this is something that you will have to practice for several days when awake before you will be able to use it at night.

Often, the thoughts that occupy our minds when we are trying to go to sleep are of worries and concerns. Or the mind may be full of all the ways we see our lives "not to be working." This imagery practice can help counter this by helping you cultivate a sense of safety and serenity that is conducive to rest. The invitation is to create an image of a serene and safe place—such as a beach, since that is a place that many people find comforting and relaxing. Or maybe it's a favorite vacation spot, a peaceful fishing spot, a cold night by a fireplace with a loved one, or a park where you go to relax—any of those might work better for you. Or think of an activity that you enjoy or would like to do more often. Activities that are soothing, relaxing, or enjoyable work best. Another possibility is something you can do endlessly, such as floating down a river. You could choose something that has continuous movement downward, paralleling the idea of "falling asleep." Whatever you use, it has to be relaxing for you, yet vivid enough to fill up your conscious mind.

Your image can be an actual scene or activity, or one that is completely made up, or a combination. It does not matter, as long as it is relaxing for you. Use a whole, vivid scene, but keep it slowly moving, maintaining calmness and serenity. Use as many of your senses as possible.

The instructions for the imagery practice are below, followed by an example of an imagery scene (after Krakow and Neidhardt, 1992).

PLEASANT IMAGERY FOR INSOMNIA

Practice this imagery exercise for five minutes once or twice during your waking hours for several days. When you get very good for a few practice sessions in a row (although you do not have to be perfect) at holding the "image" in your mind and are able to return to it quickly when your mind drifts then, *and only then,* are you ready to use it at night. (The whole process may not work well if you try to use it before you have reached this level of proficiency.)

Procedure: We will describe just what constitutes an image in a bit, but first, we need to describe the method for developing its strength in your mind.

Arrange yourself in a quiet place, uninterrupted, for ten minutes. Use the first few minutes to think about what you are about to do and to get into a comfortable, relaxing position (sitting, reclining in recliner, or lying, knees bent over a pillow and a pillow under head for comfort). When you are ready to begin practicing the image, set a timer (use a kitchen timer, the alarm on your watch or smart phone, or equivalent) for five minutes (or more if you like) and close your eyes. Keep your eyes closed and practice reliving the image in your mind until the timer tells you that the practice time is up. Slowly and calmly, but vividly, recall your chosen image. Pause between individual elements of the image so that you go at a relaxing pace, but add a new element before it all gets boring and your mind is likely to wander. Try to use all your senses as much as you can when doing this. Overall, the whole thing should flow smoothly. When the practice time is up, use the remaining time to reflect on how things went.

Some people make a point of memorizing their image before beginning this practice, but others read it as they are practicing for the first few sessions. Still others make a recording of the image to which they can listen. However, don't use it at night until you are familiar enough with it that you can recall it on your own. Playing recorded scenes can be especially helpful if you are having problems with achieving or maintaining the image. However, it is better to not play the recording when trying to get to sleep; better to rely on your own mind for this. Regardless of how you do it, you will find that you will memorize the image quickly. Also, be aware that you do not have to know it perfectly. It is okay if you skip something, add something, or take things out of order.

If something else enters your mind while practicing or using imaging at night, don't get upset. It's a natural tendency for this to happen. Acknowledge that it happened, and then *calmly* return to the image. You can do this even if a negative thought or image intrudes. It's like wandering off the trail on a hike because you noticed something interesting. You just need to return to the trail and continue the hike.

SAMPLE IMAGE: A PLEASANT BEACH SCENE

I'm standing on a little hill looking down at a beautiful beach. PAUSE. I notice the waves gently rolling in. PAUSE. The rhythmic sound of waves is soothing. PAUSE. I feel a pleasant gentle breeze from the water. PAUSE. The sea air smells so good and fresh. PAUSE. The sun soothingly warms my face. PAUSE.

I casually walk through the sand to the water's edge. PAUSE. I slip off my beach shoes. PAUSE. The warm sand feels good on my bare feet. PAUSE. I slowly stroll along the beach. PAUSE. The waves alternately wash up, then gradually recede. PAUSE. There are interesting shells being exposed by the waves. PAUSE. A wave gently washes over my feet; the cool water feels good. PAUSE.

Out on the water, the sun makes delightful glistening patterns on the waves. PAUSE. There are several beautiful sailboats gently pushed by the wind. PAUSE. Now I hear several sea gulls overhead. PAUSE. I look up and see the sea gulls as they glide overhead. PAUSE.

As I continue to walk, I notice several large rocks looming out of the sand. PAUSE. I stop and notice interesting shapes and colors of the rocks. PAUSE. Then I comfortably lie back against one of the rocks. PAUSE. I close my eyes and enjoy all the things I have just experienced.

Notice several things about this "image." First, it is not a static image. Rather, new elements are constantly but slowly being added to it to keep it fresh and interesting. Second, it contains more than visual aspects; other sense modes are also used. It also includes action. Third, there is no hurry to get through it. It is supposed to be relaxing. Yet it moves along at a pace that keeps it interesting and fresh. The image you use should also have these characteristics.

If you have difficulty imagining a sense, such as smell, there is no need to use it. Generally, though, the more senses you can use, the easier it is to keep your entire conscious mind-space filled up and focused on the image. Keeping these words in mind might help you develop the breadth of your imagery senses: *feeling, seeing, hearing, touching, tasting, smelling.*

To develop your image, you may want to begin by simply picturing an uncomplicated but calm, beautiful scene. Keep working at it until you spend more and more continuous time on the scene. Your goal is to be able to bring up the scene at will, no matter what other thoughts or images may be trying to intrude.

Sometimes, people begin to feel like they are floating while doing imagery. That's just fine. Other sensations might be a warm tingling in your legs or hands. Or perhaps you may feel a mild heaviness. In any case, enjoy it. If it becomes too unpleasant, wiggling your toes or making a brief fist can counter these feelings.

Eventually, though, you must settle on only one image that you regularly use for the rest of your life! That allows this image to become associated with falling asleep. Because of this, you will find that you will often fall asleep within minutes after starting the image. This is less likely to occur if you have more than one image that you use. However, you do not have to be too rigid within your one image; change some details now and then, let bits of it flow where it wants to go, see some parts from a different angle, start at a different place. Overall, keep it enjoyable but calm. But with whatever changes you make over time, the image should be clearly recognizable as the one used to assist you in falling asleep.

When you see that, during your practice sessions, you have gotten better, though not perfect, in holding on to the image and being able to return to it when your mind drifts off of it, then you may start using it at night. For most people, this happens after a week or two of daily practice. As you begin to use it at night, you can reduce and eventually phase out the amount of daytime practice with it. However, if, after using it successfully at night to assist you in falling asleep, it does not seem to work during a couple of nights (a common occurrence), don't give up. Instead, you might want to return to doing some practice sessions during the daytime to strengthen your ability to hold on to the image.

Also, when first using your image at night, regular nighttime practice with it will be necessary. Try using it every night for a while, whether you need it or not, so that it becomes associated with falling asleep and returning to sleep. Use it when you first go to bed for the night or when desiring to return to sleep after waking up. When you get to the point that you keep falling asleep before you finish the image (which is desirable), then you need only use it when having difficulty falling asleep or returning to sleep.

Wow! That was a lot! Now we invite you to your daily practice of the GMATI-4 meditation.

***

When you have finished, take some time to be with yourself and note what you experienced.

Now, remembering that nonjudgment is at the heart of mindfulness, what did you notice:

- In your body?
- In your mind?
- And in your mood?

We are not done yet. In the next and final chapter, we offer you some reemphasis, elaboration, and additional suggestions.

CHAPTER 8

Good Night

Continuing to Sleep Well and What to Do from Here

And so we've come to the end of this four-week journey together. You have learned a lot and have developed many skills to cultivate mindfulness and get better rest. In addition, you may have noticed that even if you are not sleeping as easily or as well as you like, you can accept this with less struggle and discomfort. That, in itself, is an incredible benefit. The less you struggle, the more peaceful your repose will be, and that *will* lead you to better sleep.

You've learned many foundational mindfulness practices, you've learned about sleep, and you've been cultivating a more compassionate relationship with yourself. You started because you were fed up with not being able to sleep the way you would like to. The suffering that came from insomnia led you here. You may have encountered ideas and practices that were familiar, new, different, or paradoxical. You learned that the best way to get some sleep was to give up trying so hard to get to sleep. You've learned about your mind and its own particular flavor of resistance. You've learned about the influence of your thoughts and emotions on your body, and how your body sensations influence your thoughts and emotions. You've seen what conditions create an experience of ease and peace, and you've seen what conditions lead to agitation and frustration. And you've learned that you can influence those conditions by where you place your attention and by what attitude you bring to any given moment. You've learned a lot!

It's not easy to develop a new daily habit of meditation. But, as you may have discovered, the payoffs can be pretty significant. You've been encouraged to meditate every day in order to train and strengthen your mindfulness muscle, and we encourage you to continue meditating every day. To inspire yourself to keep up your practice, remember that when you are meditating, you are giving your parasympathetic nervous system (otherwise known as the "relaxation response") a workout—or really a "work-in." The more we "exercise" it through meditation during the day, the more it can be activated and create an internal state of relaxation both day and night. That relaxation response is critical to being able to sleep well.

There is a story of a meditation student going to a teacher and asking, "Teacher, how long should I meditate every day?" The wise teacher responded, "If you have the time, meditate for one hour a day. If you don't have time, meditate for two hours per day." What we understand from this story is how much we need to bring balance to our lives, using an alternative mode of being to the chronic activation of busyness, the frenetic energy of modern life, and the mind's habit of negatively ruminating. We need to frequently be in a mode where we are compassionately engaging with ourselves and the present moment just as it is, with no need to get anywhere else, fix anything, or be any different than we are right now. A mode of true wholeness and rest. We all need that. And if you are struggling with not being able to rest through sleep, you need it even more.

You have a number of guided meditations you can use to continue your practice. You can go back through each of the GMATI meditations week by week, or you can stay with one that you found really resonated with you. Also, there are many options beyond this book that can help you deepen your meditation practice. You can enroll in a mindfulness-based stress reduction class in your area, or even sign up for one online. You can also look for a mindful self-compassion class if you want to delve more into that aspect of practice. (You can find local classes or online classes at the centerformsc.org website.) You can also use one of the many mindfulness apps that are available now. (Look for ones we recommend in the Resources section at the end of the book.) Whatever you do, commit yourself to making mindfulness a part of your daily life! Your mind, body, and heart will thank you for it!

GMATI Review

First, here are some general GMATI themes to remember:

- The key to GMATI is to change your relationship with your thoughts and emotions rather than trying to directly change those thoughts and emotions. The majority of your sleeplessness comes from your continued struggle with and attempts to avoid poor sleep, rather than from the poor sleep itself.

- Begin to notice if you are "trying" to sleep. If you notice you are, accept it and then let it go. Instead, *allow* sleep to happen.

- Begin to notice if you are making judgments about being awake (for example, thinking "I'm awake and this is bad"). Accept that that thought is there and then let go of your judgments.

- Remember that the work you are doing can take time. Therefore, be patient.

- If you had a "bad night," accept how you feel the next day. If you are sick or have a cold, you tend to be accepting of yourself: telling yourself that your day might not be as productive, or that you may not feel as well. In the same way, if you have a bad night's sleep, try not to put too much pressure on yourself the next day.

Now it's time for you to take steps to maintain and enhance what you have learned to do, reviewing what we have done together week by week:

In Week 1, we discussed how the struggle with insomnia worsens insomnia and wastes a lot of energy. We then said that mindfulness can help, and the GMATI-1 practice guided you through an initial mindfulness meditation exercise. The mindfulness meditation focused on simply *being aware.*

In Week 2, we emphasized how *acceptance* of your sleep as it is can help break the vicious cycle of trying unsuccessfully to control insomnia. We introduced you to the next level of GMATI meditation.

In Week 3, we emphasized the value of *letting go* of what your sleep is like and the emotions you experience because of poor sleep. Acceptance and letting go are the two important supporting components of this mindfulness meditation after being aware. You were then given the third level of GMATI meditation to practice.

In Week 4, you were encouraged to experience the rest that can come from being in the present moment just as it is. You also learned ways you can at times carefully use mindfulness at night to assist the GMATI meditation you do during the day in ways that can bring ease into your mind and heart and help to support yourself when you are not sleeping. The theme for the week was about developing *confidence,* both in your ability to sleep and in your development of mindfulness. We realize, however, that you, like many others, may from time to time experience a bout of poor sleep in the future and may need a quick refresh of the components of the GMATI program to get back on track. The following box is exactly that.

Checklist of GMATI Tools to Help You Sleep Better:

Chapter 1	
✓	Understanding Stress
✓	Styles of Thinking
Chapter 2	
✓	What Mindfulness Is
Chapter 3	
✓	What Normal Sleep Is
Chapter 4—Week 1	
✓	GMATI-1 recording
✓	Establishing a Practice
✓	Foundational Attitudes for Mindfulness Practice
✓	Reactions or Observations People Have When They Begin Meditating
✓	Weaving Mindful Awareness into Your Everyday Activities
✓	Putting Yourself on Pause
✓	Three-Minute Breathing Space
✓	Grounding
Chapter 5—Week 2	
✓	*Allowing* What Your Sleep Is Like
✓	GMATI-2 recording
✓	Mindful Stretching
✓	Diaphragmatic Breathing
✓	Affectionate Breathing
✓	Self-Compassion
✓	Self-Compassion Break
✓	Mountain Imaging

	Chapter 6—Week 3
✓	GMATI-3 recording
✓	Being Mindfully Aware of Your Thoughts
✓	Dealing with Emotions
✓	Additional Mindful Stretching
✓	RAIN: Recognize, Allow, Investigate, Non-identification.
✓	Striving, Disillusionment, Radical Acceptance
✓	Combating FOMO (Fear of Missing Out)
	Chapter 7—Week 4
✓	GMATI-4 recording
✓	Loving-Kindness Meditation
✓	Mindful Meditation at Night
✓	Shutting Off Thoughts During the Night
✓	Gratitude, Inner Smile, Loving-Kindness, Soothing Touch
✓	Pleasant Imagery for Insomnia

Relapse Prevention

In the spirit of turning toward life at it is, it's really important to honestly acknowledge that even though you may have just made great gains to improve your debilitating poor sleep, you, like most people, will probably run into a time when your sleep again begins to give you problems. This does not mean that your chronic insomnia has returned. Often, this occurs because of a life event. You need to be prepared so that a transient bout of poor sleep does not become prolonged insomnia. So let's take some time to look at some approaches for relapse prevention. "Don't let the small burning embers of transient insomnia accelerate into a blaze."

Our memories are not as accurately enduring as we typically imagine. It can be helpful to have a written record of what your sleep was like and what helped you to sleep better. Thus, the first thing we suggest is for you to write your responses now to the following questions, so you can review your answers in the future as needed.

1. How did your difficulty with sleep develop?

2. What kept your sleep difficulty going?

3. What have you learned about sleep, especially your sleep?

4. What else did you learn during the course of therapy that was helpful?

5. What were your most unhelpful thoughts and beliefs about your sleep?

    What are better alternatives to these unhelpful thoughts and beliefs?

6. What were your most unhelpful behaviors?

    What are better alternatives to these unhelpful behaviors?

7. How will you build on what you have learned? (Set goals to ensure maintenance of progress.)

If, in the future, it seems like your sleep is deteriorating, keep in mind that you mastered insomnia before, and you can master it again. First review your answers to the above questions. If that is not enough, you can do the following:

1. Try to avoid, as much as possible, conditions in which insomnia and use of sleeping pills are likely to occur.

2. Don't compensate for sleep loss by sleeping in or excessive napping.

3. Review what was shown earlier in this chapter, namely the general GMATI "themes to remember," what you have done week by week when first doing the GMATI sequence, and specific parts of the GMATI program.

4. If the insomnia persists beyond a few days, ask yourself the following and make the changes necessary: What have I been doing well to help me sleep? What am I now having difficulty with? What can I change to improve my sleep?

More on Working with Thoughts

We spent a lot of time over these past four weeks learning how to work with thoughts in meditation. This is really important, because most often it's the tone, style, and intensity of thoughts that shape how we are experiencing our lives and ourselves at any given moment. You can't control which thoughts come into the mind, but you can influence how they affect you by changing your relationship to them. Here are just a few more ideas and ways to do just that.

The Practice of "De-Literalization" and "De-Fusion"

It is all too easy to take our thoughts as absolute, literal truth. Sometimes they are, but frequently enough, they can be on a continuum ranging from only partially true to totally false. Problems occur because when we take them as literally true, we can get caught up with them and disruptively dwell on them. This is also true of how we sometimes deal with emotions. Thoughts and emotions can seem real, but are not necessarily reality. They are not always what they say they are, even if they seem to be.

In reading this book and practicing through the weeks, you've already learned how to use the sensations in the body that tend to accompany strong emotions. Likewise for thoughts with strong emotional content. You were shown how to do this by "labeling" them so that you can pay attention to your emotional experiences and honor them without needing to dwell on what's happening or getting tied up with them. Because when you see thoughts and emotions as *just what is happening in the mind at the moment,*" you can let them go more easily.

A related but stronger thing you can do is *de-literalize* your thoughts and emotions—mindfully experiencing them like any other ongoing experience by objectively describing and naming them. For example, instead of thinking, "I cannot sleep," you might instead think, "I am having the thought that I cannot get to sleep now." Or "I sometimes have a problem sleeping" instead of "I'm a hopeless insomniac." Another way is to welcome the thought by saying something like, "Hello, sleepless night thought," or "Here is that 'another poor night' thought."

Another way to de-literalize an emotion is to "physicalize" it. See it as an object with a specific shape and color that is located in or near your body. For example, you might see frustration with your sleep as a spiky red ball that is sitting on your chest.

When we take our thoughts and emotions literally, we tend to view them as describing our entire self, as if they are who we are. This can leave us feeling despondent. But when we de-literalize them, they are perceived as being only a part of us—if they are anything at all. They are manageable and we can let them go rather than being overwhelmed by them.

De-fusion is a related component. Fusion means getting caught up in our thoughts or buying into them and allowing them to dominate our behavior, whether we believe the thought or not. De-fusion means separating or distancing from our thoughts—letting them come and then go—instead of continually being caught up in them. Another way of looking at this is to "unhook" our thoughts and feelings from our actions when they are not helpful.

Imagine you are in a boat and you are holding on to a bag full of heavy belongings. Suddenly, the boat capsizes and you are being pulled under by the bag. What can you do? If you decide to let go of the bag, you can get to the surface of the water and save energy to swim to safety. It is the same with thoughts that are dragging you down: just let go of them.

A good way to defuse is to write down the thought, then notice that all that is there is just a string of words. Or try repeating a word such as "insomniac" out loud as rapidly as you can for half a minute. When you are done, you probably will note that the word loses its strength and its hold on you.

Of course, your mindfulness practice will help you create an open and curious state of mind, where you can really take hold of some of these tools.

Mindfulness Revisited

We started this book with a chapter defining what mindfulness is and isn't. You have had four weeks of practice, and so it's now time to revisit that definition. Mindfulness is "the awareness that arises when we pay attention, on purpose, in the present moment and nonjudgmentally." As you may have discovered in your own practice of meditation, the impact from developing mindfulness has the potential to go far beyond just your struggle with insomnia. The development of mindfulness can touch all aspects of life and is ultimately in the service of overall self-knowledge, wisdom, and compassion.

Self-Knowledge

Without self-awareness or self-knowledge, we have little hope of making conscious decisions about how we engage in our lives. A lack of self-awareness leaves us perpetually acting out of unconsciously acquired habits of both mind and behaviors. And these may or not be very helpful. Self-knowledge offers us a lifelong friendship with ourselves and a relationship that can grow as we age. Spiritual teacher and medical intuitive Carolyn Myss defined consciousness once in a retreat as "knowing why we act, think, speak, and even pray as we do." As we come to intimately know ourselves, we can become our own inner ally. We can gain insight and perspective on our past and present and how we want to move into our future.

Wisdom

It is from the nonjudgmental appraisal of things that we come to know their true nature. This is the cultivation of wisdom. We come to know life on its own terms. We discover that every moment we experience is a composite of conditions. This—and all of our subsequent and past moments, with all their thoughts, body sensations, feelings, and emotions—is as it is because it can't be otherwise. That's nature. If I have a garden where I plant potatoes, it would be foolish to expect corn to grow instead. Corn can't grow because the conditions for its growth aren't there.

So we learn that "accepting the moment" is simply accepting that every moment is an expression of nature, of the conditions that are currently operating. Now, being part of nature means that it is also subject to change. Nothing that exists in nature is static. Nature is process oriented. Conditions change. This is likewise true for thoughts, body sensations, feelings, and emotions. Every element of a moment is moving through a process of change. Agitation, restlessness, and sleeplessness—like any experiences—come to the body or mind, and if we feed them with resistance, they grow. If we don't, they naturally turn into something else.

Compassion

When we come to understand the constantly changing nature of things and that everything is moving through a process, we realize that there is not some other solid preferred place we need to strive for, no other fixed way we need to be, and nothing we need to force ourselves into or grasp after. The constant pressure to make ourselves be different from how we are at any given moment leads to a world of suffering. Yet it is also completely human for us to keep trying.

254

This is the exquisite tenderness of the human condition—to exist in these polarized conditioned ways of being, knowing that things are impermanent and yet continually striving to hold on to idealistic visions of how we think things should be. When we really feel into this, this vulnerability and tenderness that we all share, then compassion for ourselves and our condition naturally arises. Compassion to accept ourselves as we are. To accept the moment as it is and to move forward in our lives with an open heart. Compassion gives courage and strength to live these lives of ours with all of the messiness that goes along with being human.

Summary

In the first chapter of this book, we shared with you a few examples of people who were struggling with insomnia and sought out mindfulness. You may have seen some similarity with your own experience in those examples. During the last four weeks you have developed your own "story" for your mindfulness journey. You may feel like you've come a long way, or perhaps you feel like you're still at the very beginning but that you've gotten some traction. Regardless of where you are, you are in exactly the right place. You can only be where you are, and hopefully you've been able to taste the possibility of compassionate acceptance. Now that we've come to the end of the book, we want to share what those individuals had to say after learning mindfulness and how they were able to apply it to their lives and their sleep:

"I can't believe how much I was beating myself up for things in my body that were actually perfectly normal. I really see how much anxiety I was causing for myself!" This is what Cynthia reported after learning both mindfulness and self-compassion. "Now, when I wake up I say to myself, 'It's okay, sweetheart. This is normal and you don't need to fight it.' This has been a life changer for me."

Sam (who was recovering from cancer and dealing with a lot of chronic pain) called after he had been practicing mindfulness for two weeks. "I can't believe it!" he exclaimed. "I was able to sit free of pain for a whole thirty minutes while doing the meditation, and I even was able to fall asleep last night." His voice revealed that he was crying a little bit as he was saying these. "I just needed to call and express my gratitude," he said.

What Alex said on the last day of an eight-week MBSR class has stayed with us for years: "For a long time, I've been so freaked out by my work and the economy I've been terrifyingly convincing myself I'm going to end up homeless. Now I think, 'Well, I probably won't end up homeless, but even if I do, I'll be a lot happier than I was before I started this class.' My blood pressure is down and I'm sleeping a whole heck of a lot better!"

We've come now to the end. May your experience of practicing mindfulness through the GMATI approach grant you peace, rest, and ease of well-being! We wholeheartedly appreciate your spending the time you have reading this book and practicing GMATI and all the meditations and suggestions. May you discover the beauty of a relationship with yourself, and may that relationship result in an increase of wisdom and compassion that bring you deep rest and joy in your life!

APPENDIX

Additional Tools That Can Help If You Need Them

Bringing Awareness to Behaviors or Activities That Can Help GMATI Work Better

Although the goal of GMATI is not trying to directly fix your sleep, but allowing GMATI meditation to do it indirectly for you, there are some things you can to do for your sleep to assist what GMATI is doing. Just be sure that you do them with this attitude in mind. Otherwise, they could hinder rather than help your sleep.

HAVE THE BED = SLEEP (NOT WAKE)

- Use the bed and bedroom only for sleep and not for anything that requires being awake, such as reading, watching TV, using your phone, solving problems with your bed partner, planning, worrying (pleasurable sex is an exception).

- Avoid looking at the clock when you are having trouble sleeping. Move the clock so that you cannot easily peek at it from your bed, because seeing the time when not sleeping often causes anxiety.

- Avoid sleeping anywhere except your bed.

- If you are not sleepy at bedtime, wait to go to bed until you feel sleepy or delay bedtime, but for no more than an hour.

- Avoid lying in bed "just to rest."

- You may stay in bed when not sleeping as long as you remain calm and relaxed. You might want to say to yourself, "I can't sleep now, so I might as well enjoy the time rather than struggle to sleep."

PREPARE THE BEDROOM

- Have a comfortable bed.

- Bedroom should be comfortably dark (some people like a night light, others total darkness) and quiet.

- Bedroom temperature should be comfortable (usually a few degrees lower than daytime temperature).

PREPARE FOR BEDTIME

- Begin to "unwind" about an hour before bedtime; avoid activating or arousing behaviors; keep lights dim.

- Have a relaxing bedtime ritual (listening to soft music, taking a warm bath, praying, doing light reading, and so forth) that you do about the same time every night for ten or twenty minutes before lights-out time.

TRY TO DO THESE THINGS

- Exercise regularly (midafternoon or early evening is best; not close to bedtime if it hinders your sleep).

- Get up at about the same time every day (that is, do not sleep in).

- Eat a healthy diet on a regular schedule of meal times (less saturated fat and less sugar, but more fiber and somewhat more protein has been shown to benefit sleep).

- Avoid large meals before bedtime, but (this is optional) consider a small, light snack before bed or when awake during the sleep period.

AVOID THESE THINGS

- Trying to sleep rather than allowing sleep to happen. (GMATI will do this for you.)

- Some people may need to avoid too much caffeine during the day, and especially several hours before bedtime.

- Don't use alcohol to get to sleep, because it interferes with good sleep.

- Reduce nicotine use near bedtime.

- Limit napping to one midafternoon nap per twenty-four hours and for no longer than twenty or thirty minutes.

Sleep Efficiency and Sufficiency

Let's take a direct look at the efficiency of your sleep and how much sleep is really sufficient for you. Despite popular notions, not everyone actually needs seven or eight hours of sleep—this is just an average; for some, six hours is necessary, but for others, it is nine or even a bit more. Sleep need is largely determined by genetics. But regardless of individual sleep need, everyone benefits from sleeping efficiently. So first, let's explore sleep efficiency.

Your Sleep Efficiency

Good sleep efficiency simply means that your sleep period consists of a lot of sleep with little time awake. (The sleep period is the time between when you intend to go to sleep and when you get out of bed for the day.) Nobody is perfectly sleep efficient. It always takes some time to first get to sleep, time to get back to sleep after waking up during your sleep period, and, sometimes, time awake before getting out of bed for the day. But with good sleep efficiency, these awake times are minimal (a total of about sixty minutes or less (up to ninety minutes or so in the elderly) during an eight or nine-hour sleep period). Although there is a method of precisely determining sleep efficiency, for practical purposes when you are doing GMATI, if you are satisfied that you spend most of the sleep period asleep (realizing that there will be some time awake), then consider that you have good sleep efficiency.

Your Sleep Need

So back to your individual sleep need. As of yet, there is no known sleep lab assessment, brain measurement, blood test, or anything else that can determine an individual's sleep need. The only way is through self-evaluation. What you need is just enough sleep to efficiently satisfy your daily sleep drive while also getting enough to function well during the day.

If you are not getting enough sleep, you will find yourself suffering from many of the following: grumpiness, difficulty concentrating and reasoning, feeling tired, being accident prone, reduced sex drive, feeling down, forgetfulness, poor judgment, needing frequent naps, dozing off in quiet situations, and so forth. If you are trying to get more sleep than you need, you will find yourself excessively awake during the sleep period, especially toward the end of it. Unfortunately, there are other things that can make you feel and behave crappy during the day besides not getting enough sleep at night, and things that can keep you awake at night other than being in bed too long. Thus, you will also need to try to determine what these additional factors might be and try to correct them first, or at least take them into account when trying to determine your optimal sleep period.

So where does this leave you? If you are now sleeping efficiently and sufficiently because of your GMATI practice and are functioning well during the day, then all you need to do is to continue to meditate with a GMATI recording or some other mindfulness meditation. However, if your sleep does not seem efficient or sufficient even though it has improved with GMATI, you may need to do one of the following:

If It Seems That Your Sleep Efficiency Is Low, Then Do the Following:

(You may want to defer doing this until you are satisfied that your GMATI practice has improved your sleep.)

Determine just how much time you really need to spend in bed to get the sleep you need by first gradually reducing how much time you are spending in bed by delaying your bedtime by fifteen or twenty minutes every few nights. Keep the time that you get out of bed for the day consistent seven days a week. Continue reducing your time in bed until your sleep efficiency feels satisfactory for you.

But also pay attention to what is happening during your waking hours. Understand that when curtailing time in bed, some people initially experience some sleepiness during the day. This often only lasts a few days, but if and when it does happen, driving should be limited to only brief periods at a time and you should avoid doing anything dangerous. However, if you begin to experience continuing sleepiness or the waking problems typical of insufficient sleep (such as the ones listed in the section above), you should stop reducing your sleep period. At this point, gradually lengthen your sleep period by fifteen minutes or so every few days until your daytime is relatively free from problems of insufficient sleep.

You may need to experiment between lengthening and shortening your sleep period until you find the happy medium that is right for you of decent sleep efficiency and minimal daytime problems. Once you arrive at this compromise, plan on staying with it. But don't be in a hurry to accomplish this. Spend a few nights after you make a change just getting used to the change before you make another one. Also, it is a good idea to avoid napping while doing this procedure.

If You Feel That You Are Not Getting Enough Sleep, But the Sleep You Get Seems to Be of Good Efficiency, Then Consider the Following:

You will know that you are not getting enough sleep if you are experiencing too many waking problems associated with insufficient sleep, such as those listed above. If so, here is what you can do. (Note: Be very careful to be sure that you are sleeping efficiently and yet are not getting enough sleep. It is all too common for people with insomnia to think that "if I spend more time in bed, I am more likely to get more sleep, the sleep I need." Unfortunately, they frequently wind up spending even more time awake in bed, which actually then worsens their sleep efficiency and their insomnia. The goal is having both relatively good sleep efficiency and good functioning during the day.)

To get more sleep time while maintaining good sleep efficiency, first gradually increase how much time you are spending in bed by going to bed fifteen or twenty minutes earlier every few nights while keeping the time that you wake up and get out of bed for the day consistent every morning. Stop increasing your time in bed when you begin to experience poor sleep efficiency. It is also a good idea to avoid napping while doing this procedure.

As you are doing this, you should begin to notice fewer daytime problems due to insufficient sleep. Your goal is to settle in on a compromise between good sleep efficiency and few daytime problems. Then, plan on remaining on this schedule.

Tapering Off Sleeping Pills

It may be that you are still taking sleeping pills to help you sleep. Now that you are sleeping better because of using GMATI, you are ready to taper off of them if you want to. While GMATI can work well while you are taking sleeping medications, we think it is better, as much as possible, to be able to sleep with the resources you have inside of yourself rather than to need something external, such as sleeping pills. For a relatively few people, it may be necessary to take some kind of sleep aid because they have weak sleep drive brain mechanisms, but most of us can sleep well without them.

Quitting cold turkey does not work for a lot of people. If they have a night or two of poor sleep for whatever reason, they tend to think that forgoing a sleeping medication is not working for them, so they give up and go back to using it. In contrast, the following schedule is more effective because it has you regularly alternate between taking a lower dose with taking a full dose. Over time, the lower-dose nights become more frequent and the full-dose ones become less frequent. This tends to be more successful because if there is a night or two of poor sleep, the thought is, "This is okay because on future nights I will be able to take the full dose yet stay on the schedule." That is, people are much more likely to stay with their desire to get off of the medication. So here are the details of this more effective way to taper off of sleeping medications.

This paragraph explains what is shown in the chart below. You may want to frequently refer to it while reading this. You start by choosing a lesser amount of the medication you have been taking, such as a half dose, but it could be a smaller reduction, such as three-fourths of your usual dose, if you feel that would be more tolerable for you. Use a lower dose of it if available or split the does you are now taking. (This also might depend on the ability to split your pills. If the medication you want to stop taking is of the continuous-release form, do not split it.) If you are taking more than one drug to help you sleep, then consult with your primary care provider about which one to taper first.

During the first week, alternate a night of the lower dose (such as a half dose) with two nights of the full dose. The second week, alternate one night of the lower dose with one night of the full dose. The third week, alternate two nights of the lower dose with one night of the full dose. The fourth week, take the lower dose every night. If at this point the lower dose is still too much and you can still split it into smaller amounts, then you repeat this schedule with the current low dose assuming the role of the full dose and a new lower dose being a further fraction of the original full (such as one-fourth). However, if the current lower dose is close to zero or if it is not possible to split it further, then the new low dose becomes 0 (nothing at all).

Schedule For Tapering Off Sleeping Pills Following Successful Use Of GMATI
(Based on Lichstein et al., 2013.)

Notice: You must consult with and get permission from your primary care provider before using this plan to reduce your use of prescription sleeping pills.

Tapering schedule model where ● = the dose you currently take regularly and ◖ = usually 1/2 (or some other fraction) of that dose. Smaller steps may be better.

Day	1	2	3	4	5	6	7
	◖	●	●	◖	●	●	●
Day	8	9	10	11	12	13	14
	●	◖	●	◖	●	◖	◖
Day	15	16	17	18	19	20	21
	●	◖	◖	●	◖	◖	●
Day	22	23	24	25	26	27	28
	◖	◖	◖	◖	◖	◖	◖

Return to week 1 using the dose taken during week 4 as the new regular dose

OR

continue as shown below when your current dose is low enough that you can start tapering to nothing

Day							
	◖	◖		◖	◖		◖
Day							
		◖		◖		◖	
Day							
		◖			◖		
Day							

Use this chart to plan your taper schedule based on the drug and dose you are now using.

Night	1	2	3	4	5	6	7
Night	8	9	10	11	12	13	14
Night	15	16	17	18	19	20	21
Night	22	23	24	25	26	27	28
Night	29	30	31	32	33	34	35
Night	36	37	38	39	40	41	42
Night	43	44	45	46	47	48	49

Resources

Books and Articles

Brach, T. 2003. *Radical Acceptance: Embracing Your Life with the Heart of a Buddha.* New York: Bantam.

Brach, T. 2013. *True Refuge: Finding Peace and Freedom in Your Own Awakened Heart.* New York: Bantam.

Chodron, P. 1997. *When Things Fall Apart: Heart Advice for Difficult Times.* Boston: Shambala.

Germer, C. 2009. *The Mindful Path to Self-Compassion.* New York: Guilford Press.

Hanson, R. 2009. *The Buddha's Brain.* Oakland, CA: New Harbinger Publications.

Hanson, R. 2014. *Hardwiring Happiness.* New York: Harmony/Crown.

Kabat-Zinn, J. 1990. *Full Catastrophe Living: Using the Wisdom of Your Body and Mind to Face Stress, Pain, and Illness.* New York: Bantam Doubleday Dell.

Kabat-Zinn, J. 1994. *Wherever You Go, There You Are: Mindfulness Meditation in Everyday Life.* New York: Hyperion Press.

Knox, M., K. Neff, and O. Davidson. 2016. "Comparing Compassion for Self and Others: Impacts on Personal and Interpersonal Well-Being." Cited in K. Neff and C. Germer. 2018. *The Mindful Self-Compassion Workbook: A Proven Way to Accept Yourself, Build Inner Strength, and Thrive.* New York: Guilford Press.

Moorcroft, W.H. 2013. *Understanding Sleep and Dreaming,* 2nd edition. New York: Springer Press.

Neff, K. 2011. *Self-Compassion: The Proven Power of Being Kind to Yourself.* New York: William Morrow.

Neff, K., and C. Germer. 2018. *The Mindful Self-Compassion Workbook: A Proven Way to Accept Yourself, Build Inner Strength, and Thrive.* New York: Guilford Press.

Ong, J.C. 2017. *Mindfulness-Based Therapy for Insomnia.* Washington, DC: American Psychological Association.

Ong, J.C., R. Manber, Z. Segal, Y. Xia, S. Shapiro, and J. Wyatt. 2014. "A Randomized Controlled Trial of Mindfulness Meditation for Chronic Insomnia." *Sleep* 37: 1553–1563.

Ong, J.C., C.S. Ulmer, and R. Manber. 2012. "Improving Sleep with Mindfulness and Acceptance: A Metacognitive Model of Insomnia." *Behaviour Research and Therapy* 50: 651–660.

Sapolsky, R.M. 1998. *Why Zebras Don't Get Ulcers: An Updated Guide to Stress, Stress-Related Diseases, and Coping.* New York: W.H. Freeman.

Salzberg, S. 1997. *Lovingkindness: The Revolutionary Art of Happiness.* Boston: Shambala.

Siegel, D.J. 2010. *Mindsight.* New York: Bantam.

Segal, Z.V., J.G. Williams, and J.D. Teasdale. 2002. *Mindfulness-Based Cognitive Therapy for Depression: A New Approach to Preventing Relapse.* New York: Guilford Press.

Websites

UCSD Center for Mindfulness: health.ucsd.edu/specialties/mindfulness/Pages/default.aspx

Mindfulness-Based Cognitive Therapy: www.mbct.com

Center for Mindful Self-Compassion: centerformsc.org

Kristin Neff: self-compassion.org

Tara Brach: www.tarabrach.com

Society for Behavioral Sleep Medicine: behavioralsleep.org

American Academy of Sleep: aasmnet.org

Northern Colorado Sleep Consultants, LLC: sleeplessincolorado.com

Meditation Apps

Head Space: www.headspace.com

The Mindfulness App: themindfulnessapp.com

References

Barraclough, J. "The Importance of Imagery in Sport." believeperform.com/performance/the-importance-of-imagery-in-sport/

Brach, T. 2013. *True Refuge: Finding Peace and Freedom in Your Own Awakened Heart.* New York: Bantam.

Brach, T. 2018. "Working with Difficulties: The Blessings of RAIN." www.tarabrach.com/articles-interviews/rain-workingwithdifficulties/

Cartwright, R., A. Luten, M. Young, P. Mercer, and M. Bears. 1998. "Role of REM Sleep and Dream Affect in Overnight Mood Regulation: A Study of Normal Volunteers." *Psychiatry Research* 81: 1–8.

Clarey, C. 2014. "Olympians Use Imagery as Mental Training." www.nytimes.com/2014/02/23/sports/olympics/olympians-use-imagery-as-mental-training.html

Creswell, J.D., B.M. Way, N.I. Eisenberg, and M.D. Lieberman. 2007. "Neural Correlates of Dispositional Mindfulness During Affect Labeling." *Psychosomatic Medicine* 69: 560–565.

Garland, S., W. Britton, N. Agagianian, R.E. Goldman, L.E. Carlson, and J.C. Ong. 2015. "Mindfulness, Affect, and Sleep: Current Perspectives and Future Directions." In K. Babson and M. Feldner (Eds.), *Sleep and Affect: Assessment, Theory, and Clinical Implications* (pp.339–373). Elsevier, Inc.

Germer, C., and K. Neff. 2017. *Mindful Self-Compassion Teacher Guide.* San Diego, CA: Center for Mindful Self-Compassion.

Kabat-Zinn, J., 1994. *Wherever You Go, There You Are: Mindfulness Meditation in Everyday Life.* New York: Hyperion Press.

Krakow, B., and J. Neidhardt. 1992. *Conquering Bad Dreams and Nightmares.* New York: Berkley Books.

Lichstein, K., S. Nau, N. Wilson, R. Aguillard, K. Lester, A. Bush, and C. McCrae. 2013. "Psychological Treatment of Hypnotic-Dependent Insomnia in a Primarily Older Adult Sample." *Behaviour Research and Therapy* 51: 787–796.

Neff, K.D. (2003). "Self-Compassion: An Alternative Conceptualization of a Healthy Attitude toward Oneself." *Self and Identity* 2: 85-102.

Neff, K. 2018. "Embracing Our Common Humanity with Self-Compassion." self-compassion.org/embracing-our-common-humanity-with-self-compassion

Neff, K., and C. Germer. 2018. *The Mindful Self-Compassion Workbook: A Proven Way to Accept*

Yourself, Build Inner Strength, and Thrive. New York: Guilford Press.

Ong, J., and D. Sholtes. 2010. "A Mindfulness-Based Approach to the Treatment of Insomnia." *Journal of Clinical Psychology* 66: 1175–1184.

Sapolsky, R. 1998. *Why Zebras Don't Get Ulcers: An Updated Guide to Stress, Stress-Related Diseases, and Coping.* New York: W.H. Freeman.

Segal, Z., J. Williams, and J. Teasdale. 2002. *Mindfulness-Based Cognitive Therapy for Depression: A New Approach to Preventing Relapse.* New York: Guilford Press.

Steller, J.E., and D. Keltner. 2014. "Compassion." In M. Tugade, L. Shiota, and L. Kirby (Eds.), *Handbook of Positive Emotions* (pp.329–341). New York: Guilford Press.

Catherine Polan Orzech, MA, LMFT, has taught mindfulness since 2000. She received her initial training in mindfulness-based stress reduction (MBSR) at the Center for Mindfulness at the University of Massachusetts Medical Center, and her professional training under the direction of Jon Kabat-Zinn, and is certified to teach MBSR and mindful self-compassion (MSC). She has taught and lectured on the subject of mindfulness internationally, and was founder and codirector of the Montreal Center for Mindfulness. Catherine has been on the faculty at numerous mindfulness institutes, including Thomas Jefferson University Hospital's Myrna Brind Center for Integrative Medicine in Philadelphia, PA.; the University of California, San Francisco's Osher Center for Integrative Medicine; and the University of California San Diego's Mindfulness-Based Professional Training Institute.

Catherine is currently an instructor in the departments of psychiatry and OB-GYN at Oregon Health & Science University, where she's involved in research on mindfulness and women's health. Her program on mindful and compassionate parenting is currently the subject of research at the University of Oregon. Catherine currently lives in Corvallis, OR, where she is a marriage and family therapist in private practice specializing in mindfulness-based psychotherapy focusing on individuals, couples, and families. Find out more about Catherine at www.corvallismindfulnesstherapy.org.

William H. Moorcroft, PhD, is a registered psychotherapist; behavioral sleep medicine specialist; emeritus professor at Luther College, Decorah, IA; and founder and chief consultant at Northern Colorado Sleep Consultants, LLC, where he now specializes in treating insomnia, children's sleep problems, nightmares, and sleep problems in shift workers. He is also former director of a Sleep and Dreams Laboratory. Following earning a PhD from Princeton University, Moorcroft committed over forty-five years of his to life studying and researching sleep and dreams. During this time, he did additional sleep disorder training at the Mayo Clinic in Minnesota and Rush Medical College in Chicago, IL. He has previously authored four books, many research papers, and numerous other publications. Find out more at www.sleeplessincolorado.com.

Foreword writer **Jason C. Ong, PhD,** is associate professor in the department of neurology at Northwestern University's Feinberg School of Medicine. He is past president of the Society of Behavioral Sleep Medicine, and author of *Mindfulness-Based Therapy for Insomnia.*

MORE BOOKS *from*
NEW HARBINGER PUBLICATIONS

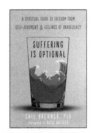
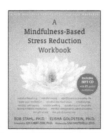
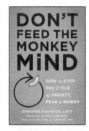
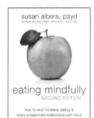
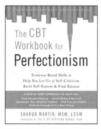
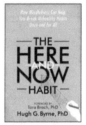
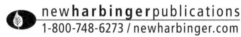

Register your **new harbinger** titles for additional benefits!

When you register your **new harbinger** title—purchased in any format, from any source—you get access to benefits like the following:

- Downloadable accessories like printable worksheets and extra content

- Instructional videos and audio files

- Information about updates, corrections, and new editions

Not every title has accessories, but we're adding new material all the time.

Access free accessories in 3 easy steps:

1. Sign in at NewHarbinger.com (or **register** to create an account).

2. Click on **register a book**. Search for your title and click the **register** button when it appears.

3. Click on the **book cover or title** to go to its details page. Click on **accessories** to view and access files.

That's all there is to it!

If you need help, visit:

NewHarbinger.com/accessories

new harbinger
CELEBRATING
40 YEARS

Back Cover Material

An Innovative Mindfulness Program to Help You Get Your Zzzs

Sleep plays a crucial role in our waking lives. When we get a good night's sleep, we wake up feeling refreshed, alert, heathier, and ready to face the day ahead. And when we don't get the rest we need, we end up tired, unfocused, grumpy, and even depressed. If you're one of countless people who suffer from insomnia and its negative effects, the soothing mindfulness practices in this book will help ease you back to truly restorative sleep.

In *Mindfulness for Insomnia,* you'll learn how to break the cycle of anxious thinking, rumination, and tension that keeps you up at night. Using the innovative four-week mindfulness protocol, you'll also uncover the emotional stresses that lie at the root of your sleep issues, and find practical mindfulness techniques to alleviate the physical and mental effects of sleep loss. Most importantly, you'll discover how to create the conditions necessary for a restful and healthy slumber, so you can feel your best and *be* your best.

"A dynamic combination of invaluable information and practical skills to support mind and body wellness."
—DIANE REIBEL, PhD, coauthor of *Teaching Mindfulness*

CATHERINE POLAN ORZECH, MA, LMFT, is a veteran mindfulness expert. She received formal training at the Center for Mindfulness at the University of Massachusetts Medical Center under the direction of Jon Kabat-Zinn, and is a certified mindfulness-based stress reduction (MBSR) instructor.

WILLIAM H. MOORCROFT, PhD, is a registered psychotherapist and behavioral sleep medicine specialist who specializes in treating insomnia. He is author of *Understanding Sleep and Dreaming.*

Made in United States
Troutdale, OR
06/03/2024

20313620R00170